Cytopathology of the Glandular Lesions of the Female Genital Tract

Monographs in Clinical Cytology

Vol. 20

Series Editor

Svante R. Orell Kent Town

Cytopathology of the Glandular Lesions of the Female Genital Tract

Matías Jiménez-Ayala Madrid
Beatriz Jiménez-Ayala Portillo Madrid

Including contributions by

Francesc Alameda Barcelona
Carmen Alvarez-Santín Montevideo
Belén Lloveras Barcelona
Dina R. Mody Houston, Tex.
Ritu Nayar Chicago, Ill.
Manuel Nevado Santos Madrid
Lara Pijuán Barcelona
Fernando Pinedo Moraleda Madrid
Maria Carmen Rodríguez Alvarez Montevideo
Volker Schneider Freiburg
Adela Sica Montevideo
Michael Thrall Houston, Tex.

170 figures, 168 in color, and 26 tables, 2011

KARGER Basel · Freiburg · Paris · London · New York · Bangalore · Bangkok · Shanghai · Singapore · Tokyo · Sydney

Monographs in Clinical Cytology

Dr. Matías Jiménez-Ayala
Instituto Jiménez-Ayala
Hermosilla 126
E-28028 Madrid (Spain)
E-Mail matiasjimenezayala@hotmail.com

Dr. Beatriz Jiménez-Ayala Portillo
Instituto Jiménez-Ayala
Hermosilla 126
E-28028 Madrid (Spain)
E-Mail beatriz@institutojimenezayala.com

Library of Congress Cataloging-in-Publication Data

Jiménez-Ayala, Matías.
Cytopathology of the glandular lesions of the female genital tract / Matías Jimenéz-Ayala, Beatriz Jimenéz-Ayala Portillo ; including contributions by Frances Alameda Barcelona ... [et al.].
p. ; cm. -- (Monographs in clinical cytology, ISSN 0077-0809 ; v. 20)
Includes bibliographical references and index.
ISBN 978-3-8055-9464-6 (hard cover : alk. paper) -- ISBN 978-3-8055-9465-3 (e-ISBN)
1. Generative organs, Female--Cytopathology. I. Jiménez-Ayala Portillo, Beatriz. II. Title. III. Series: Monographs in clinical cytology ; v. 20. 0077-0809
[DNLM: 1. Genital Neoplasms, Female--diagnosis. 2. Genital Neoplasms, Female--pathology. 3. Cytodiagnosis--methods. 4. Neoplasms, Glandular and Epithelial--diagnosis. 5. Neoplasms, Glandular and Epithelial--pathology. W1 MO567KF v. 20 2011 / WP 145]
RG107. 5. C95. J56 2011
618.1--dc22

2010041126

This publication was sponsered by

QIAGEN

Bibliographic Indices. This publication is listed in bibliographic services, including Current Contents®.

www.karger.com
Printed in Switzerland on acid-free and non-aging paper (ISO 9706) by Reinhardt Druck, Basel
ISSN 0077–0809
ISBN 978–3–8055–9464–6
e-ISBN 978–3–8055–9465–3

To Sara, for her family 'sacrifices' during her first 2 years of life and
in the hope she will be the third step in our cytopathology saga.

Contents

Preface

Following our first publication in the Karger series *Monographs in Clinical Cytology* (vol. 17), which was devoted to endometrial adenocarcinoma, we have spent the last 2 years to preparing this second volume, *Glandular Lesions of the Female Genital Tract*. We have been supported in this by series editor Dr. Svante Orell and Karger Publishers. The subject is an area in which we have wide experience and, on this occasion, we have been honored to welcome contributions from 12 international experts in the cytopathology of glandular lesions. Their writings cover the wide spectrum of this challenging subject.

Genital glandular lesions, both benign and malignant, are an attractive area of cytopathology. Malignant lesions of the endocervix and endometrium are becoming more common all the world, compared to squamous cell carcinoma. In this volume we present discussions of in situ and invasive endocervical adenocarcinoma, endometrial adenocarcinoma and endometrial hyperplasias.

Ovarian lesions focusing data obtained from intraoperative studies are considered. Other areas of the genital tract, such as the vulva and the fallopian tube, which are less common and thus have seen fewer publications, are also presented. The impact of the Bethesda System and basic and ancillary techniques in the study of glandular lesions complete our monograph.

We hope that this monograph will be useful to cytopathologists, pathologists, cytotechnologists and to students of these specialities, as it deals with the most common areas of their daily work.

Acknowledgements

Our gratitude goes to Dr. Svante Orell and to Mr. Thomas Nold for their stimulating discussions and help in the preparation of this book. Thanks also to the contributors and to the staff of the Instituto Jiménez-Ayala, with special mention to Paloma Fernandez Rueda for her dedicated and efficient secretarial work, and to senior cytotechnologist Concha Chinchilla.

Matías Jiménez-Ayala, FIAC. Instituto Jiménez-Ayala and Former Chair, Department of Cytology, Hospital Universitario Gregorio Marañón, Madrid, Spain

Beatriz Jiménez-Ayala Portillo, MIAC. Director, Instituto Jiménez-Ayala, Madrid,

Foreword

Glandular lesions of the female genital tract have always been a challenge for pathologists. The precise cytological diagnosis of these lesions is difficult because of their inherent complexity, as well as the lack of experience of many cytopathologists in this field.

This monograph brings to us an extensive review of the different glandular lesions of the female genital tract that can be recognized on cytological material. Through the different chapters, many authorities in the area show, in a very didactic way, the morphological criteria and the main differential diagnosis of several glandular lesions that will be very useful for pathologists and cytopathologists in daily practice. The 12 well-organized chapters also cover important topics in the area, such as routine and ancillary techniques for the diagnosis of glandular lesions and the 2001 Bethesda System classification of glandular lesions on cervical cytology. There are 170 figures, 168 in color, most of them of excellent quality – an important point in books dealing with morphological criteria for diagnosis. The 351 references distributed throughout the book and cited at the end of each chapter provide extensive coverage of all conditions discussed.

Some words for the editors of the monograph. For the first time in the 50-year history of the prestigious *Monographs in Clinical Cytology,* the same authors have been responsible for 2 different volumes of the series. Dr. Matias Jiménez-Ayala and Dr. Beatriz Jimenéz-Ayala Portillo were also editors of volume 17, entitled Endometrial Adenocarcinoma: Prevention and Early Diagnosis. This fact reflects the extensive experience of both editors in the field of glandular lesions of the female genital tract. As mentioned before, in this book they invited the most prestigious cytopathologists around the world with experience in glandular lesions to write, ensuring the excellent quality of the text.

In summary, this monograph is once more a valuable addition to the Karger series *Monographs in Clinical Cytology*, which is edited by Dr. Svante Orell, and I am quite sure that this book will be a practical bench resource for all professionals involved in the cytological diagnosis of glandular lesions of the female genital tract.

Fernando Schmitt, MD, PhD, FIAC
General Secretary of the International Academy of Cytology
Institute of Pathology and Molecular Immunology of Porto University, IPATIMUP
Medical Faculty of Porto University, Porto

List of Abbreviations

ACC	Adenoid cystic carcinoma
AD	Adenosis
ADSC	Adenosquamous carcinoma of the cervix
AEC	Atypical endocervical cells
AEmC	Atypical endometrial cells
AGC	Atypical glandular cells
AH	Atypical hyperplasia
AIS	Endocervical adenocarcinoma in situ
ASC-H	Atypical squamous cells, high-grade SIL not excluded
ASC-US	Atypical squamous cells of undetermined significance
ASR	Arias-Stella reaction
BGC	Bartholin gland carcinoma
BS	Bethesda System
CCA	Clear cell adenocarcinoma
CE	Cervical endometriosis
CGIN	Cervical glandular intraepithelial neoplasia
CIN	Cervical intraepithelial neoplasia
CIS	Squamous carcinoma in situ
CVS	Cervicovaginal smear
DES	Diethylstilbestrol
EA	Endocervical adenocarcinoma
EBT	Endometrial brushing techniques
EC	Endometrial cytology
EH	Endometrial hyperplasia
EIA	Early invasive adenocarcinoma
EIN	Endometrial intraepithelial neoplasia
EmA	Endometrial adenocarcinoma
EMBT	Endocervical mucinous borderline tumor
EN	Endometrioid neoplasia
EP	Endocervical polyp
FNAC	Fine needle aspiration cytology
FT	Fallopian tube
FTC	Fallopian tube carcinoma
GCC	Glassy cell carcinoma of cervix
GCT	Granulosa cell tumor
HC2	Hybrid Capture 2
HPV	Human papillomavirus
HSIL	High-grade squamous intraepithelial lesion
IMBT	Intestinal mucinous borderline tumor
IUD	Intrauterine device
LBP	Liquid-based preparation
LUS	Lower uterine segment
MA	Mucinous adenocarcinoma
MBT	Mucinous borderline tumor
MC	Metastatic carcinomas
MGH	Microglandular hyperplasia
MT	Metastases
NOS	Not otherwise specified
PB	Psammoma bodies
PD	Paget's disease
PH	Papillary hidradenoma
PHGC	Post-hysterectomy glandular cells
RVF	Rectovaginal fistulaes
SA	Serous adenocarcinoma
SBT	Serous borderline tumor
SCC	Squamous cell carcinoma
SIL	Squamous intraepithelial lesion
SPC	Serous papillary carcinoma
SSPC	Serous surface papillary carcinoma of the ovary
TM	Tubal metaplasia
VC	Vulvar carcinoma
VGA	Villoglandular adenocarcinoma
VIN	Vulvar intraepithelial neoplasia
VSIL	Vulvar squamous intraepithelial lesion

List of Authors

Francesc Alameda, MIAC. Department of Pathology, Hospital del Mar, Barcelona, Spain. Officer, Spanish Society of Cytology (Chapter 12).

Carmen Alvarez-Santín, MIAC. Former Professor of Pathology, University of Montevideo, Uruguay. Secretary General, Latin American Society of Cytology (Chapter 8).

Matías Jiménez-Ayala, FIAC. Instituto Jiménez-Ayala, Madrid. Former Chair, Department of Cytology, Hospital Universitario Gregorio Marañón, Madrid, Spain. Former President of the International Academy of Cytology (Chapters 5, 6, 7, 9, 10, 11).

Beatriz Jiménez-Ayala Portillo, MIAC. Director, Instituto Jiménez-Ayala, Madrid, Spain (Chapters 3, 5, 10, 11).

Belén Lloveras, Department of Pathology, Hospital del Mar, Barcelona, Spain (Chapter 12).

Dina R. Mody, MD. Professor of Pathology and Laboratory Medicine, Weill Medical College of Cornell University. Director of Cytology Laboratory and Fellowship Program, The Methodist Hospital, Houston, Tex., USA (Chapter 2).

Ritu Nayar, MIAC. Professor of Pathology and Director of Cytopathology, Northwestern University, Feinberg School of Medicine, Chicago, Ill., USA (Chapter 2).

Manuel Nevado Santos, MIAC. Chair, Department of Pathology, Hospital Infanta Cristina, Parla, Madrid, Spain (Chapter 1).

Lara Pijuán, Department of Pathology, Hospital del Mar, Barcelona, Spain (Chapter 12).

Fernando Pinedo Moraleda, Chair, Department of Pathology, Hospital Universitario Fundación Alcorcón, Madrid, Spain (Chapters 1, 9, 10).

Maria Carmen Rodríguez Alvarez. Chair, Dermatopathology Area, Department of Pathology, Centro Hospitalario Pereira Rosell, Montevideo, Uruguay (Chapter 9).

Volker Schneider, FIAC. Head, Pathology Laboratory, Freiburg, Germany. Former Secretary General, International Academy of Cytology (Chapter 4).

Adela Sica. Department of Pathology, University of Montevideo, Montevideo, Uruguay (Chapter 8).

Michael Thrall, Assistant Professor, Department of Pathology and Laboratory Medicine, Weill Medical College of Cornell University, The Methodist Hospital, Houston, Tex., USA (Chapter 2).

Chapter 1

Cytopathological Techniques for the Diagnosis of Glandular Lesions of the Genital Tract

1.1. Introduction

In spite of increasing standardization, some variations in preparation, fixation and staining methods still occur between different laboratories. A clear understanding of these techniques is mandatory to optimize the quality of cytological smears.

Many ready-to-use commercial kits are now available that produce reliable and consistent staining; indeed, automation in various forms has improved efficiency in the cytopathology laboratory. New liquid-based technologies can produce monolayered cell samples, eliminate background and provide optimal concentration of epithelial cells. Some of these are based on vacuum filtration, others on density gradient centrifugation. In addition to conventional staining techniques, they also allow human papillomavirus (HPV) DNA testing, histochemistry, immunocytochemistry, and other special studies. The basic techniques of cytopreparation are summarized in this chapter with an overview of laboratory processing.

1.2. Fixation [4]

A fixative suitable for cytological specimens must preserve the morphology of the cells as well as their cytochemical and immunocytochemical properties. The most commonly used fixative in cytology laboratories is 95% ethanol. Eighty percent isopropanol, 100% methanol, or 95% denatured alcohol are also suitable. Smears have to be fixed in alcohol for about 10–15 min. Prolonged fixation does not significantly affect subsequent studies. Slides can remain in alcohol for hours or days if the staining process has to be deferred (fig. 1.1).

Different coating alcohol-based fixatives can be sprayed over fresh smears with excellent results. In addition to fixation, these products provide a protective layer over the smear when drying. They are the fixatives of choice when the smears have to be sent to the laboratory from a distant collecting point. Prior to staining coated smears, the product must be removed by dipping the slides in 2 changes of 95% ethanol for 5–10 min each.

Carnoy's fixative – composed of 60% ethanol, 30% chloroform and 10% glacial acetic acid – may be preferable for bloody samples. The slides are placed in the fixative for 3–5 min and then dipped in 95% ethanol for 10 min. By hemolyzing the erythrocytes, Carnoy's solution facilitates the study of diagnostic cells.

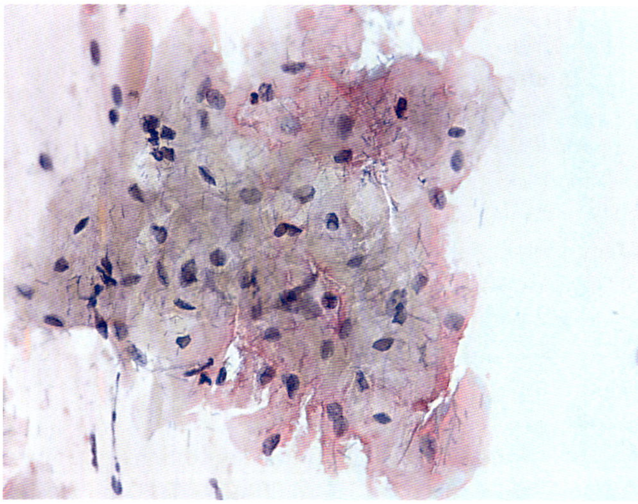

Fig. 1.1. The choice of an appropiate fixative is critical for an optimal evaluation of the smear. Pap, 400×.

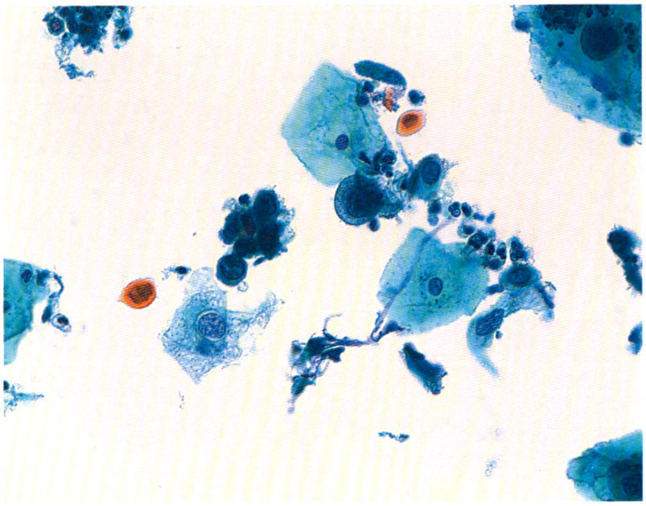

Fig 1.2. Keratinized and non-keratinized small-sized cervical cells with highly displastic featuresin a case of high-grade squamous intra-epithelial lesion. Pap LBP, 400×.

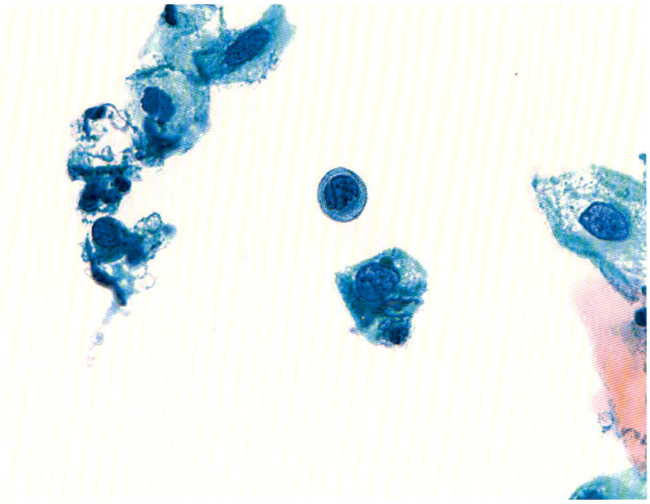

Fig. 1.3. Differences between conventional and liquid-based cytology: highly displastic cells in liquid-based cytology show lesser nuclear hyperchromasia, while nuclear irregularities are more obvious. Pap LBP, 400×.

The 2 currently FDA-approved liquid-based preparations (LBP) for cytology are SurePath® and ThinPrep®. The fixatives used in these systems are ethanol- and methanol-based, respectively. The exact composition of either solution is not publicized. In both techniques, samples are collected using a specially designed brush, which is suspended in the fixative solution immediately after completion of sampling. This permits fixation as well as mid-term conservation of samples. Optimal preservation and morphological quality are assured with both methods. Examples of liquid-based preparations can be seen in figures 1.2 and 1.3.

1.3. Staining [4]

Papanicolaou (Pap) staining is the universally accepted method for gynecological samples. It was first published in 1942 and subsequently modified in 1954 by Papanicolaou. Many variants of this technique have been developed by other authors. In summary: hydration, dehydration, bluing solutions, hematoxylin (for nuclear stain), Orange G and EA solution (for cytoplasmic and nucleolar stain) result in cellular transparency and prepare the cell sample for the final steps of mounting and coverslipping. The type of EA solution may be varied to best suit different samples. For gynecologic samples, EA solution 36 or 50 are recommended, since they result in a more contrasted cytoplasmic counter-staining. EA solution 50 is available commercially, as is Orange G. Commercially prepared reagents provide more reproducible and consistent results, and are time-saving.

Automated staining procedures can also be used to make the technique more efficient, to avoid human mistakes, and achieve optimal staining results. If imaging systems are used, reagents and standard staining protocols developed by the manufacturer must be utilized.

Mounting and cover-slipping can be done manually or by automated procedures. Automated cover-slipping machines are safer and time-saving, facilitating the work of the technicians. Machines using a special resin-coated film eliminate the need for traditional coverslips and mounting media. However, 24 × 60 mm glass coverslips are the best choice, providing better protection and preservation of smears. Glass coverslips are also preferred when using imaging systems, reducing slide rejections and imaging 'events'. The 'cornflake artifact' is frequently encountered in screening cervical smears (fig. 1.4).

It is important to establish an appropriate schedule for systematic replacement of staining reagents adapted to the volume of preparations processed. As a general rule, alcohols used for the dehydrating and rehydrating process, EA solution and Orange G stains should be replaced weekly. Bluing solutions have to be changed daily. Xylene should be replaced when it appears tinted. Hematoxylin does not need to be replaced. It is sufficient to refill the recipients with a small amount equivalent to loss due to evaporation.

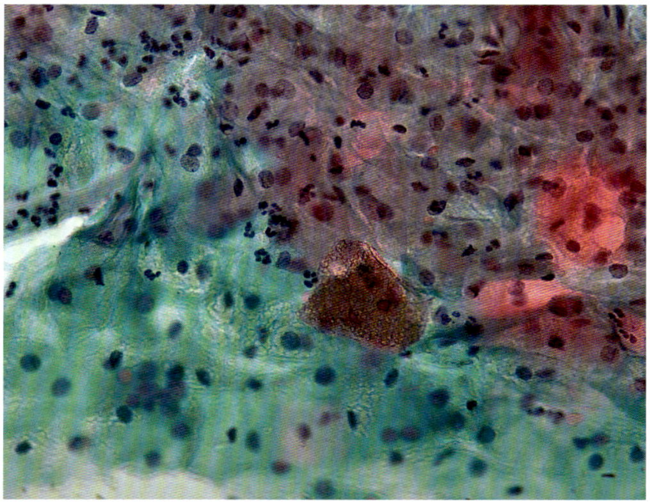

Fig. 1.4. Coverslipping artifact ('cornflake artifact'): This brown artifact over a squamous cell is air trapped when xylene is evaporated before applying mounting media. Pap, 400×.

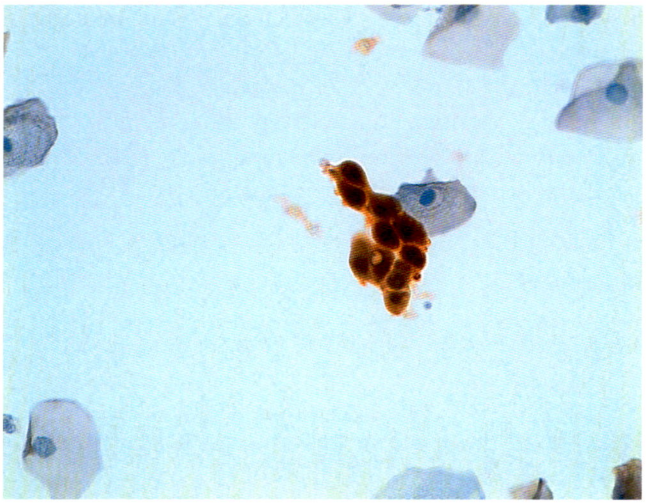

Fig. 1.5. Typical uniform nuclear and cytoplasmatic expression of p16 in a group of cells with dysplastic features. p16, 400×.

1.4. Special Techniques [1–3, 5–7]

Potentially, a vast array of additional techniques may be applied to routine cytopathology (histochemistry, morphometric techniques, electron microscopy, immunocytochemistry, cytogenetics, flow cytometry, 'in situ' hybridization and PCR).

Congo Red staining of a fine needle aspiration sample of abdominal adipose tissue for detecting amyloidosis, use of Perls stain to detect occult alveolar hemorrhage, Giemsa stain to better visualize *Leishmania* and other parasites, or Grocott silver stain for fungus or *Pneumocystis carinii* in respiratory secretions are examples of histochemistry applied to cytology. These stains are not frequently used in gynecological cytology. In general, the staining methods can be applied as in histopathology with few or only minor modifications. Optimal results are achieved relatively easily.

The use of immunocytochemistry in diagnostic cytopathology has added a new dimension to cytological diagnosis. In this context, cyto-cell blocks offer great advantages. Cell blocks are processed using the same protocols as for histological sections and allow many different immunostains to be done on paraffin sections. Tissue architecture can also be evaluated. However, most of times it is not possible to make cell blocks from gynecological samples. As a good alternative, thin-layer LBP also result in good preservation of antigenicity – even after long-term storage – and allow a number of different stains to be made. Finally, exfoliative cell samples fixed in alcohol, specially collected for immunohistochemistry processing, may be appropriate. Routinely stained and mounted cytological preparations can be reprocessed and used for immunocytochemistry, although results are poorer.

Many monoclonal and polyclonal antibodies are suitable for cytology, with variable sensitivity and specificity. Their immunoreactivity may vary and is highly dependent on the fixation process. Positive and negative controls must be performed with each test sample.

False positive results can be caused by inappropriate fixation, drying artifacts, low antibody's specificity, cytomorphological misinterpretation, and the presence of necrotic cells and debris. False negative results may be due to poor antigen preservation (fixation), insufficient antigen retrieval, inadequate antibody concentration, or insufficient representative cells in the sample.

Of course, clinicopathologic correlation is vital to achieve a correct diagnosis.

In gynecological samples, overexpression of p16, determined by immunohistochemistry, is strongly related with high-risk HPV infection (97% in high-grade squamous intraepithelial lesions; fig. 1.5). Wilms' tumor gene product (WT1) is a sensitive and specific marker for serous carcinoma of ovarian surface epithelial origin. Sox-9 expression can be used for ovarian tumors (positive in 44% of Sertoli cell tumors, 65% of well-differentiated endometrioid carcinomas, 39% of Sertoli-form endometrioid carcinomas and 10% of carcinoid tumors). Hepatocyte nuclear factor-1β is positive in ovarian clear cell carcinomas, and negative in mesothelial cells and non-clear cell adenocarcinomas.

The clinical importance of molecular diagnosis of diseases and prediction of therapy response is rapidly expanding. Consequently, molecular techniques are becoming an increasingly important part of cytopathology.

Fluorescence in situ hybridization, PCR and hybrid capture system can be applied in cytological samples for the detection of HPV DNA.

Other techniques (morphometry, electron microscopy, flow cytometry) are applicable to cytological preparations but are only rarely used in clinical practice.

References

1 Abati A, Fetsch P, Filie A: If cells could talk: the application of new techniques to cytopathology. Clin Lab Med 1998;18:561–583.

2 Bubendorf L, Grote HJ, Syrjänen K: Molecular techniques; in Bibbo M, Wilbur D (eds): Comprehensive Cytopathology, ed 3. Philadelphia, Saunders Elsevier, 2008, pp 1071–1090.

3 Chivukula M, Dabbs DJ: Immunocytochemistry; in Bibbo M, Wilbur D (eds): Comprehensive Cytopathology, ed 3. Philadelphia, Saunders Elsevier, 2008, pp 1043–1069.

4 Keebler CM, Facik M: Cytopreparatory techniques; in Bibbo M, Wilbur D (eds): Comprehensive Cytopathology, ed 3. Philadelphia, Saunders Elsevier, 2008, pp 977–1003.

5 Osamura RY: Molecular cytopathology: a new era of clinical cytology. Acta Cytol 2009;53:245–246.

6 Raab SS: Factors affecting the adoption of new cytology technologies. Diagn Cytopathol 2004;30:105–106.

7 van Hoeven KH, Fitzpatrick BT, Bibbo M: Update of immunocytochemistry in cytopathology. Pathol Annu 1995;30:245–247.

Chapter 2

2001 Bethesda System Classification of Glandular Lesions on Cervical Cytology

2.1. Introduction

As a screening test for squamous cell carcinoma of the cervix and its precursors, the Pap test has been at the core of the most effective cancer screening program ever devised. The Pap test was not designed to sample and diagnose glandular lesions/adenocarcinomas of the cervix/uterus [8]. Because of its location, squamous pathology is easier to sample and is also more readily identified cytologically than glandular abnormalities. However, with improvement in sampling techniques, including brooms and brushes, as well as better recognition of endocervical abnormalities by cytologists, these lesions may be detected by the Pap test. Since the relative as well as absolute incidence of endocervical adenocarcinoma has been rising in proportion to squamous cell carcinoma in screened populations, it is important for those involved in cervical cancer screening to be aware of the cytological criteria for diagnosis of glandular abnormalities and the subsequent management of such abnormalities detected by cervical cytology [21].

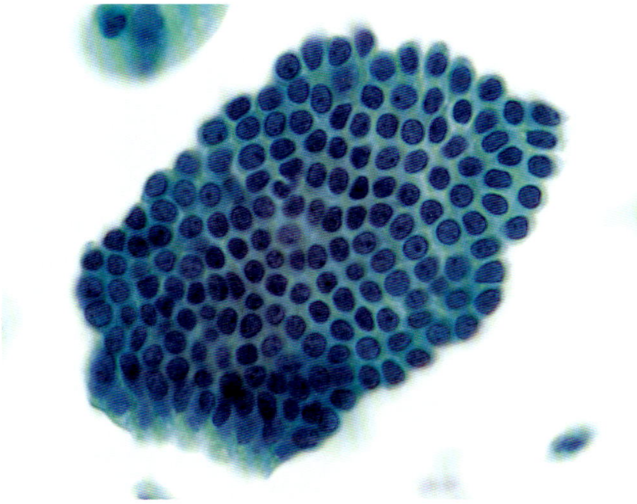

Fig. 2.1. Normal endocervical cells. The cells form regular honeycomb sheets and have a columnar configuration. LBP, SurePath.

Glandular/metaplastic cells in cervical cytology preparations are used as a marker for sampling of the transformation zone or squamocolumnar junction where squamous dysplasias typically arise. Most glandular cells sampled in Pap tests are readily classified as normal endocervical cells by their characteristic appearance: columnar cells with basal round nuclei and abundant vacuolated apical cytoplasm with groups having a 'picket fence' appearance when laid out horizontally relative to the slide surface and a 'honeycomb' structure when oriented en face (fig. 2.1). Large 3-dimensional groups from aggressive sampling are also readily identified in most instances by the presence of smooth and continuous borders on the cluster surface. Under adequacy criteria in the 2001 Bethesda system (BS) for reporting cervical cytology, the absence of an endocervical component does not limit specimen interpretation, but it is mentioned as a quality indicator that may result in an earlier than routine follow-up [17]. There is no convincing evidence that absence of an endocervical component increases the false negative rate of a Pap test.

The BS provides a framework for reporting glandular abnormalities in a uniform manner [17] (table 2.1). This allows for standardization of not only the nomenclature but also for uniform follow up. For example, in the United States, the American Society of Colposcopy and Cervical Cytology (ASCCP) has published management guidelines

Table 2.1. Outline of 2001 Bethesda System categories

Epithelial Abnormalities: Glandular
Atypical glandular cells
Atypical endocervical cells
Not otherwise specified
Favor neoplastic
Atypical endometrial cells
Atypical glandular cells
Not otherwise specified
Favor neoplastic
Endocervical adenocarcinoma in situ
Adenocarcinoma
Endocervical
Endometrial
Extrauterine
Not otherwise specified
Other
Endometrial cells present in a woman ≥40 years of age

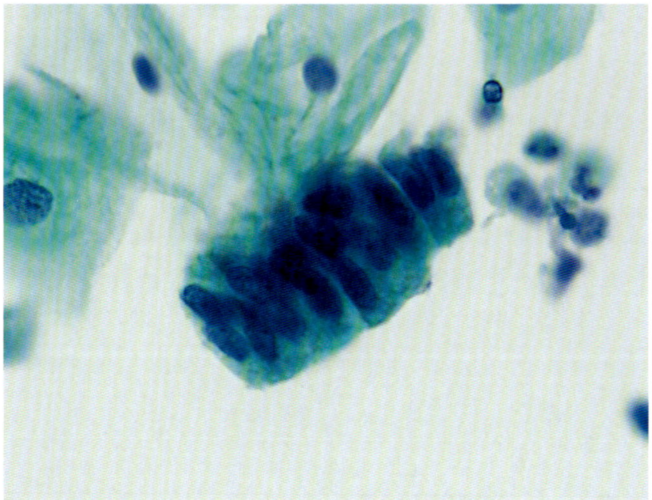

Fig. 2.2. Atypical endocervical cells, NOS. This aggregate has ambiguous atypical features that may be either reactive or AIS. LBP, SurePath.

for abnormal cytology and histology that correlate with Bethesda interpretation categories [23]. A number of significant changes in terminology and reporting were introduced in the 2001 version of the BS, to reflect the better understanding of glandular neoplasia since the previous version in 1991. The hope is that by standardizing terminology and criteria the effectiveness of cervical cytology as a detection method for glandular lesions will increase.

2.2. Glandular Epithelial Cell Abnormalities

2.2.1. Atypical Glandular Cells

The term 'atypical glandular cells' (AGC) in the 2001 BS has replaced the 1991 Bethesda terminology of 'atypical glandular cells of undetermined significance' (AGUS or AGCUS). It encompasses a wide variety of findings that fall between easily recognized reactive or reparative changes and easily recognized adenocarcinoma. AGC represents an interpretive gray zone reflecting uncertainty on the part of the cytologist about the presence or absence of a significant abnormality. As such, it is the glandular equivalent of the category 'atypical squamous cells of undetermined significance' (ASC-US) that was also first introduced in the 1991 BS. Indeed, the 2001 name change was prompted by confusion with ASC-US due to the similarity of the terms [18].

The BS provides site-specific criteria for the identification of AGC and recommends designation of a likely site of origin (endocervical versus endometrial) whenever possible to help guide the diagnostic work-up. Thus the subcategories 'atypical endocervical cells' (AEC) and 'atypical endometrial cells' (AEmC) have been included in the nomenclature. However, in some instances the origin cannot be confidently ascertained, in which case the general term AGC may be used.

Another important change from the 1991 BS is the elimination of the qualifier 'favor reactive' for AGC. Instead, atypia that can confidently be attributed to reactive changes should be interpreted as negative. Only cases in which there is uncertainty about neoplasia should be classified as AGC. Those cases with a high index of suspicion can be characterized as 'favor neoplastic' with the rest being 'not otherwise specified' (NOS). This distinction is not recommended for AEmC due to the difficulty in making this judgment in endometrial cells.

2.2.2. Atypical Endocervical Cells

AEC, like their normal counterparts, demonstrate a columnar cell configuration. The deviation from normal is recognized architecturally by increased cell crowding, loss of mucin and nuclear overlap in strips and sheets of cells. Helpful but variable nuclear features include nuclear enlargement (3–5 times the size of a normal endocervical cell), anisonuceosis, hyperchromasia, nucleoli, and rare mitoses. Increased nucleus-to-cytoplasm ratio and distinct cell borders are other features commonly seen in AEC (fig. 2.2). The use of the subcategory 'favor neoplastic' may be justified when observed cell

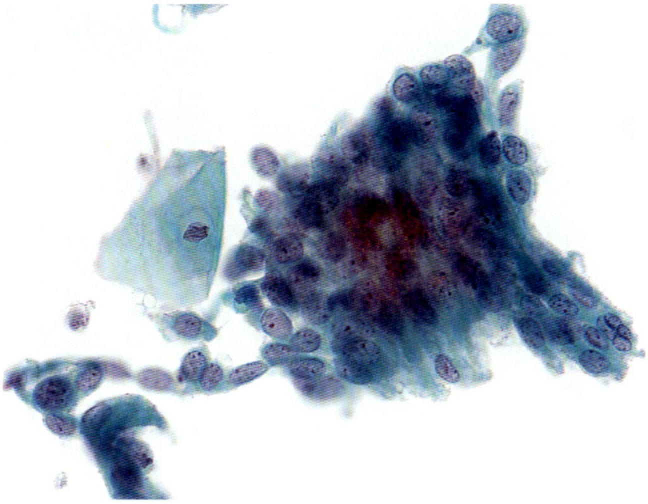

Fig. 2.3. Atypical endocervical cells, favor neoplastic. This cluster has atypical features suggestive of AIS but not entirely diagnostic. LBP, ThinPrep.

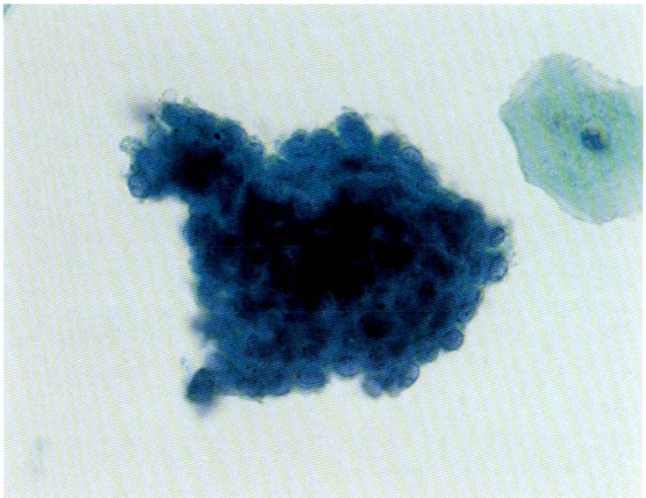

Fig. 2.4. Normal endometrial cells. The cells are in a tightly packed ball and have high nucleus-to-cytoplasm ratio. LBP, ThinPrep.

Table 2.2. Criteria for atypical endocervical cells

Not otherwise specified
Should be present:
Sheets and strips with some cell crowding and nuclear overlap
Increased nucleus-to-cytoplasm ratio (may have fairly abundant cytoplasm)
Some variation in nuclear size and shape
May or may not be present:
Nuclear enlargement (up to 3–5 × normal)
Mild hyperchromasia
Nucleoli
Rare mitoses
Distinct cell borders
Favor Neoplastic
Should be present:
Sheets and strips of cells with nuclear crowding and overlap
Enlarged nuclei with hyperchromasia
Increased nucleus-to-cytoplasm ratios (with diminished cytoplasm)
May or may not be present:
Cell groups show feathering or rosette formation
Occasional mitoses
Ill-defined cell borders

changes include focal features suggestive of adenocarcinoma in situ (AIS), more markedly abnormal instances of the other features already listed, or loss of clear cell borders (fig. 2.3). Groups tend to be more rounded and 3-dimensional in liquid-based preparations (LBP), sometimes making the application of these criteria more challenging, especially in the central portions of clusters [9] (table 2.2).

2.2.3. Atypical Endometrial Cells

The criteria for AEmC are generally even more difficult to apply [13]. Normal endometrial cells appear in tight clusters with irregular outlines, have high nucleus-to-cytoplasm ratios, dark nuclei, and irregular nuclear borders (fig. 2.4). In short, normal endometrial cells have many of the features considered 'atypical' in other settings. Some criteria that may be helpful in identifying AEmC have been put forward. Nuclear enlargement is the most distinctive marker. Architecturally, AEmC groups are often fairly small (5–10 cells). Mild hyperchromasia may be seen, as well as small nucleoli. Vacuolated cytoplasm and loss of clear cell borders may also indicate atypia (fig. 2.5). Normal endometrial cells may show greater nuclear pleomorphism, appear more hyperchromatic, and have small nucleoli in LBP Pap tests (table 2.3).

No specific criteria have been listed in the BS for AGC not of endocervical or endometrial origin. In general, the principle is the same regardless of the suspected origin of the cells: suspicious changes not definitive for adenocarcinoma should be called AGC (fig. 2.6, 2.7). This will prompt an appropriate workup to determine whether an underlying high-grade lesion or malignancy in fact exists.

Assigning an interpretation of AGC requires careful separation of truly atypical cells from a number of benign mimics [22]. The list of possible causes includes many simulators of endocervical carcinoma including repair, tubal metaplasia, microglandular hyperplasia, and endocervical

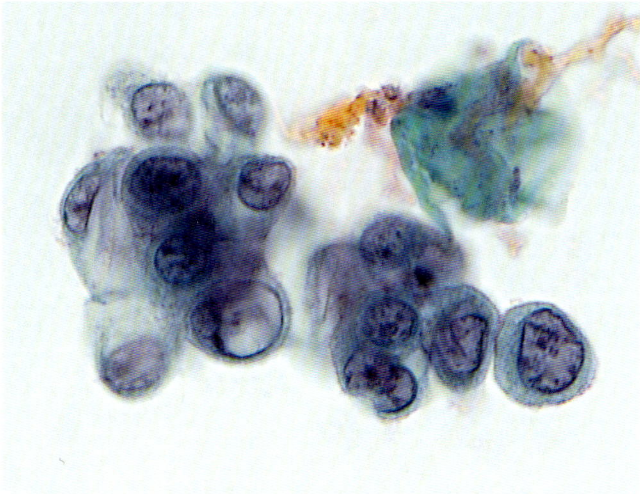

Fig. 2.5. Atypical endometrial cells. These clusters have the configuration of endometrial cells but have atypical features raising the possibility of malignancy. LBP, ThinPrep.

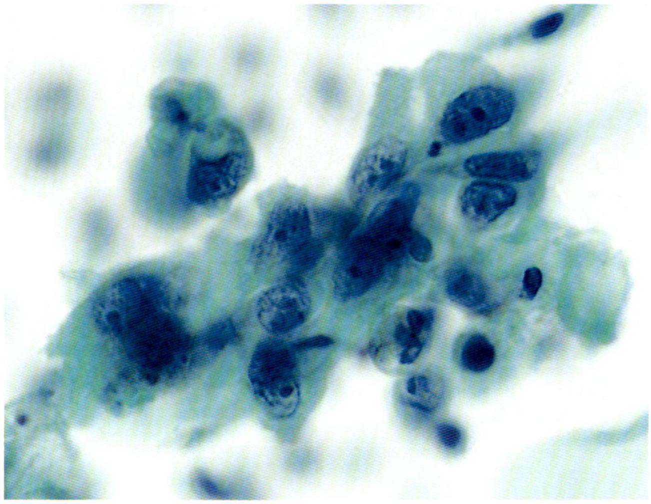

Fig. 2.6. Atypical glandular cells, NOS. This cell group appears glandular and has atypia but cannot be assigned to a more specific category. LBP, SurePath.

Table 2.3. Criteria for atypical endometrial cells

Should be present:
Cells occur in small groups (5–10 cells per group)
Nuclear enlargement (often slight)
Ill-defined cell borders
May or may not be present:
Mild hyperchromasia
Small nucleoli
Vacuolated cytoplasm

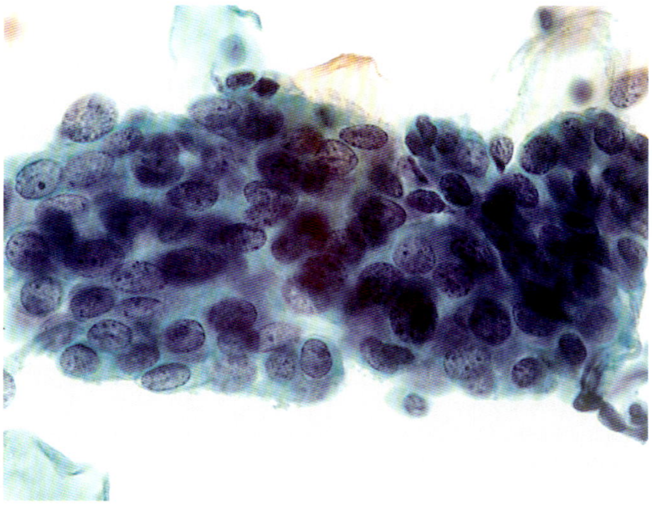

Fig. 2.7. Atypical glandular cells, favor neoplastic. This gland-like aggregate has nuclear atypia suggestive of either endocervical or endometrial neoplasia. LBP, ThinPrep.

polyps. Endometrial malignancy may be simulated by benign changes including intrauterine device effects, Arias-Stella reaction, and direct sampling of lower uterine segment. Radiation changes may also cause difficulty, especially since they are typically found in women with a previous history of malignancy. All of these potential mimics have characteristic features that, when present and supported by appropriate history, make possible confident identification of these processes as benign. Considering these alternative explanations for atypia will prevent many unnecessary interpretations of AGC and spare excessive patient work-up. Unfortunately, there will always be some examples of these changes that cannot be dismissed, justifying the equivocal category of AGC.

The possibility of a high-grade squamous intraepithelial lesion (HSIL) involving endocervical glands must also be kept in the differential diagnostic consideration of glandular atypia. Crowded groups of HSIL (severe dysplasia/carcinoma in situ) may be difficult or impossible to distinguish from true glandular atypia, especially when nucleoli are present.

2.3. Endocervical Adenocarcinoma in situ

In the 2001 Bethesda terminology, AIS, which is the glandular equivalent to HSIL (severe dysplasia/carcinoma in situ/CIN3) in the squamous classification scheme, is a distinct

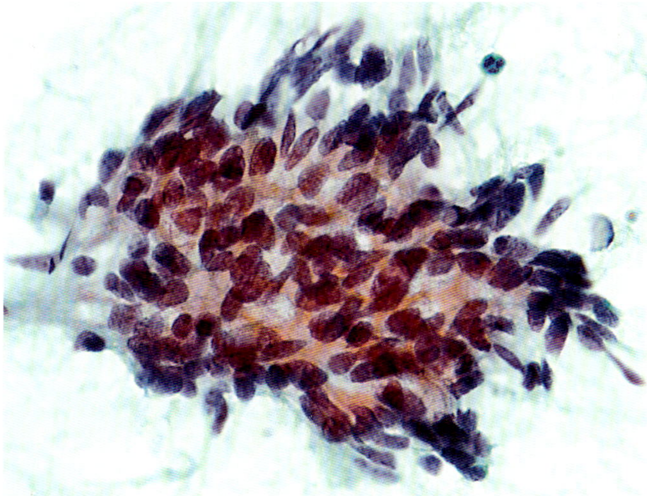

Fig. 2.8. Adenocarcinoma in situ. An illustration of the classic AIS architecture and nuclear changes in conventional smears.

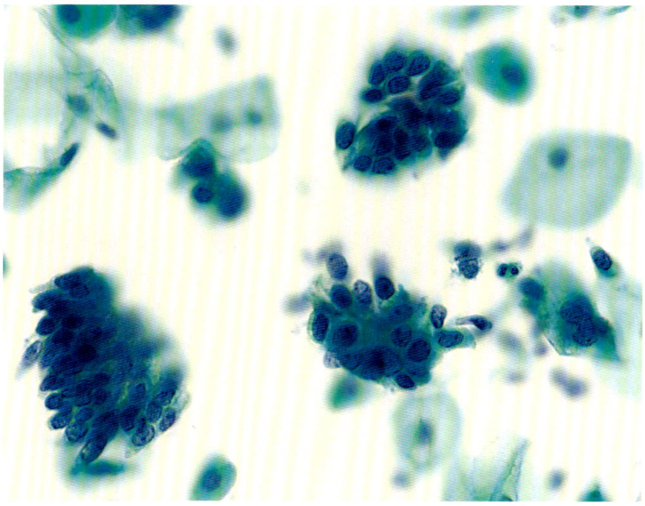

Fig. 2.9. Adenocarcinoma in situ. Feathering (bottom left) and rosette formation (center) are easily seen in this example of AIS. LBP, SurePath.

interpretive category. Like HSIL, it is thought to represent the high-risk, pre-invasive lesion before invasive carcinoma in the spectrum of intraepithelial neoplastic progression attributable to human papiloma virus (HPV). Distinctive cytological features make it possible to specifically identify this entity on cervical cytology in many cases, though some have equivocal features leading to an interpretation of 'AGC, favor neoplastic'.

Criteria for the cytological interpretation of AIS that are very useful include: nuclear feathering, pseudopalisading and rosette formation of endocervical cells. While these findings are not specific, any time they are seen AIS must be strongly considered. Feathering describes an architectural arrangement corresponding to the stratification observed histologically: nuclei and wisps of cytoplasm protrude individually from cell clusters in a palisaded arrangement giving an appearance reminiscent of the wingtip feathers of a gliding bird of prey. Rosettes, like those seen in other organs, consist of rounded clusters of cells with a distinct central clearing. Although full-blown rosettes may be absent, areas of nuclear crowding and overlap in sheets, clusters, or strips of cells suggest the same process of disorderly growth (fig. 2.8).

Additional criteria, while less evocative, must also be considered when contemplating an interpretation of AIS. Most important are nuclear features. Nuclear enlargement with elongation is as characteristic of AIS as feathering or rosetting. Nuclei are hyperchromatic with coarsely granular chromatin; mitoses and apoptotic bodies are frequent. Cytoplasm is reduced with variably decreased mucin production in most cases. Nucleoli are not usually seen. Examination of the background may reveal coexisting squamous dysplasia or a tumor diathesis suggesting the possibility of an invasive carcinoma.

In liquid-based Pap tests, more rounded, denser, more smooth-edged balls of cells tend to predominate in cases with AIS [9]. Nuclear features may also be less readily recognizable, as chromatin may be finer and more open. Nucleoli or chromocenters are more often seen in AIS cells on LBP Pap tests (fig. 2.9). Single cells may appear, a feature rarely seen in conventional smears. The 'bird tail', a feature sometimes seen in AIS on LBP, especially SurePath Pap tests, is a short strip of cells with stratified nuclei and a fanned-out appearance much narrower at the base than the surface (fig. 2.10; table 2.4).

2.4. Adenocarcinoma

Invasive adenocarcinoma may be primary to the cervix, invasive into the cervix from the endometrium or adjacent organs, or metastatic to the cervix from distant sites. Depending on the site of origin, the cytological features may differ. However, malignant cells, insofar as they are malignant, share many similar features that cytologists are very familiar with: nuclear enlargement, nuclear pleomorphism, dark and clumpy chromatin with parachromatin clearing, macronucleoli, numerous mitoses, apoptosis, and

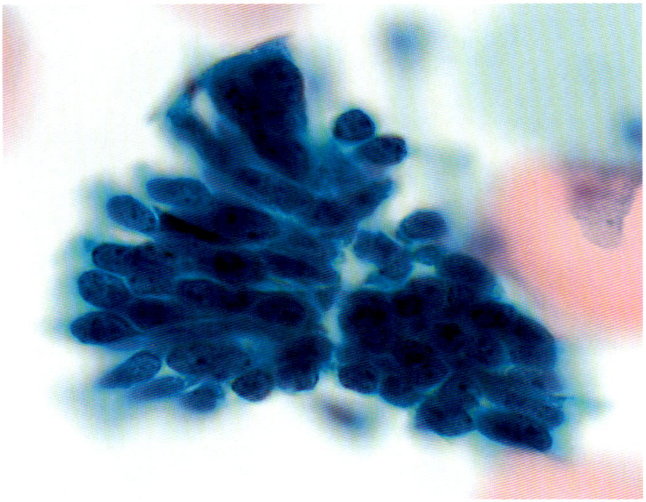

Fig. 2.10. Adenocarcinoma in situ. An example of the 'bird tail' structure of AIS seen in liquid-based preparations. SurePath.

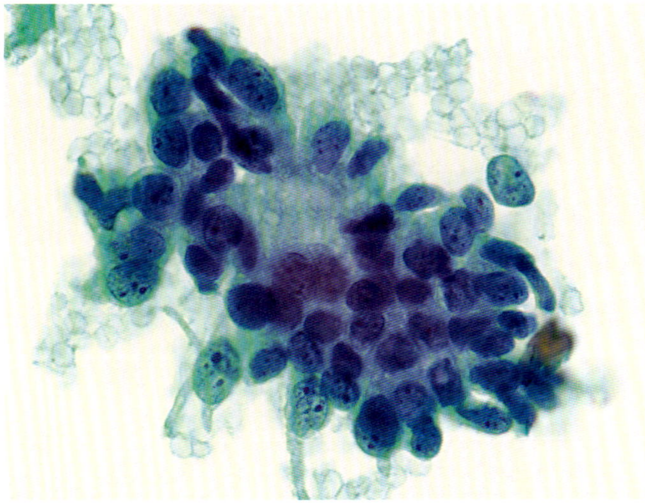

Fig. 2.11. Endocervical adenocarcinoma. This cluster has an architecture resembling AIS but also has more marked nuclear atypia and a diathesis. LBP, ThinPrep.

Table 2.4. Criteria for endocervical adenocarcioma in situ

- Sheets, clusters, strips, or rosettes of cells with nuclear crowding and overlap
- Feathering (palisaded cell clusters with protruding nuclei and cytoplasm)
- Nuclear enlargement with anisonucleosis, elongation, and stratification
- Nuclear hyperchromasia with evenly dispersed coarsely granular chromatin
- Mitosis and apoptotic bodies are common
- Some cells show a definite columnar arrangement
- Inconspicuous or small nucleoli
- Increased nucleus-to-cytoplasm ratios with decreased cytoplasm and mucin
- Clean background (diathesis or inflammation suggests invasion)
- Abnormal squamous cells may also be present

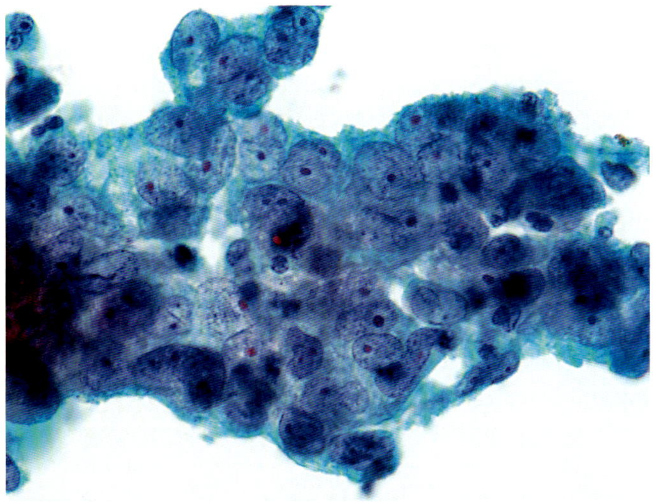

Fig. 2.12. Endocervical adenocarcinoma. This cluster retains nuclear features recognizable as endocervical despite malignant atypia. LBP, ThinPrep.

background diathesis. Recognition of overt malignancy is generally less difficult than the identification of borderline atypia. The BS offers specific criteria for the 2 most commonly encountered types of adenocarcinoma in the cervix.

Endocervical adenocarcinoma shows features of overlap with AIS. It also coexists with squamous dysplasia or malignancy in many instances, and may be the less readily apparent component [20]. Cellularity is typically high. The malignant cells usually retain the columnar morphology of their benign precursors and also tend to recapitulate glandular sheets and clusters, though in a haphazard manner. Single dyscohesive cells may be present. Cytoplasm is typically finely vacuolated (fig. 2.11). LBP tend to result in more frequent 3-dimensional clusters of cells and may make tumor diathesis less apparent. Nuclei may also be less strikingly hyperchromatic due to a more vesicular chromatin pattern, though clumping and irregularity will remain (fig. 2.12; table 2.5).

Endometrial adenocarcinoma (EmA) presents additional challenges. It arises further from the site of Pap test sampling, thus usually resulting in fewer cells and more degenerative changes in the tumor cells that are present. Tumor diathesis, often described as watery due to its finely granular

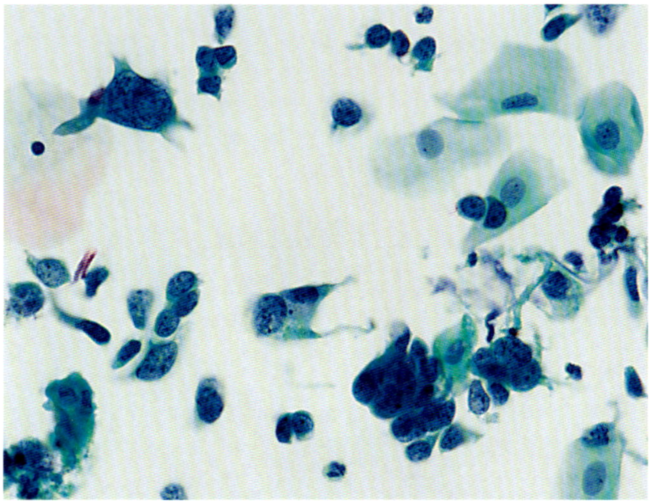

Fig. 2.13. Endometrial adenocarcinoma. A moderate-power view of endometrial adenocarcinoma shows high cellularity and markedly atypical cells. LBP, SurePath.

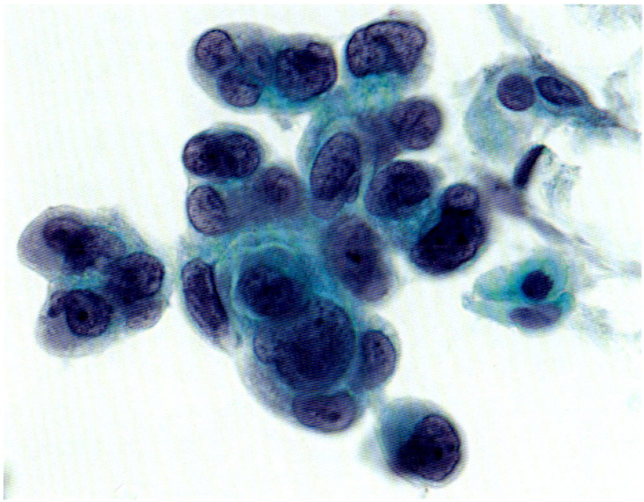

Fig. 2.14. Endometrial adenocarcinoma. This higher power view shows atypical and dyscohesive cells that retain recognizably endometrial features. LBP, SurePath.

Table 2.5. Criteria for endocervical adenocarcinoma

- Abundant abnormal cells, typically with columnar configuration
- Enlarged, pleomorphic nuclei with irregular chromatin, parachromatin clearing, and nuclear membrane irregularities
- Single cells, 2-dimensional sheets, 3-dimensional clusters, and syncytial aggregates are commonly seen
- Macronucleoli may be present
- Cytoplasm is usually finely vacuolated
- Tumor diathesis may be present
- Abnormal squamous cells may be present

Table 2.6. Criteria for endometrial adenocarcinoma

- Cells occur singly or in small, tight clusters
- Nuclear enlargement (varies by grade from slight to marked)
- Variation in nuclear size and loss of polarity
- Nuclear hyperchromasia with irregular chromatin and parachromatin clearing (especially high-grade tumors)
- Nucleoli (varies by grade from small to large)
- Scant cyanophilic cytoplasm that may be vacuolated or contain engulfed neutrophils
- Watery (finely granular) diathesis may be present

texture, may not be readily apparent. Architectural changes seen histologically, particularly glandular overgrowth, are frequently the first indication of malignancy with only subtle accompanying cellular atypia that may not be detectable cytologically.

The BS criteria for EmA include: nuclear enlargement, anisonucleosis, loss of nuclear polarity, nuclear hyperchromasia, chromatin clumping with parachromatin clearing, nucleoli, and vacuolated cytoplasm (fig. 2.13). However, all of these features may be subtle in low-grade adenocarcinomas and may be so marked as to obscure the tumor origin in high-grade tumors (fig 2.14). Intracytoplasmic neutrophils are sometimes a striking finding in EmA. Their presence should prompt consideration of malignancy but they can be seen in benign processes. As with endocervical adenocarcinoma, LBP tend to make endometrial clusters more 3-dimensional, cause nuclei to appear more vesicular, and dilute any diathesis that may be present (table 2.6).

Specific criteria for other adenocarcinoma types occasionally encountered in Pap tests have not been detailed in the BS. However, a comment should be made regarding serous papillary adenocarcinoma. The characteristic findings include papillary structures with dense 3-dimensional collections of high nucleus-to-cytoplasm ratio cells. The nuclei, if not obscured by crowding or degenerative changes show marked enlargement, hyperchromasia with chromatin clumping, and prominent nucleoli (fig. 2.15, 2.16). Psammoma bodies may also be present. Although psammoma bodies seen on a Pap test should prompt consideration of serous papillary adenocarcinoma, they may also be seen in benign conditions (fig. 2.17).

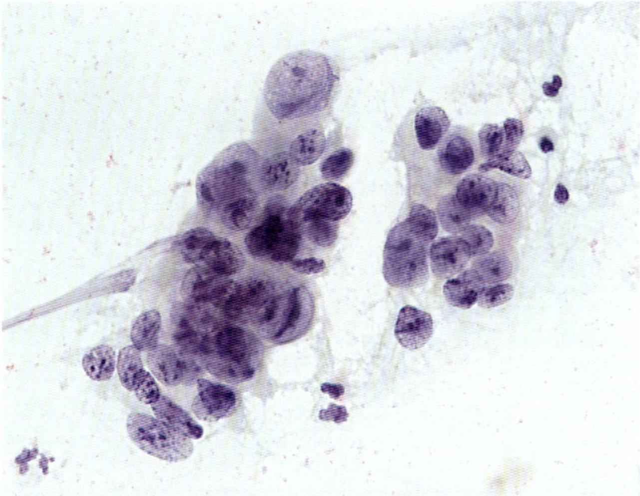

Fig. 2.15. Adenocarcinoma, NOS. This serous papillary carcinoma is easily recognized as malignant. Conventional smear.

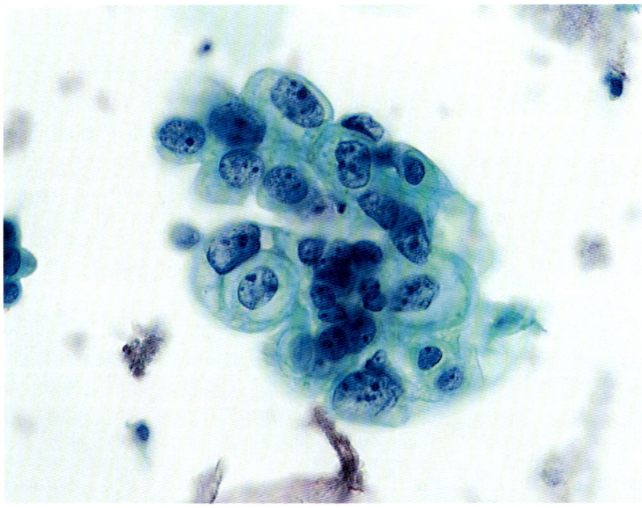

Fig. 2.16. Adenocarcinoma, NOS. A serous papillary carcinoma with obvious malignant features as seen in a liquid-based specimen. LBP, SurePath.

2.5. Other

2.5.1. Endometrial Cells in Women ≥40 Years of Age

Another change related to glandular cells introduced in the 2001 BS was the introduction of an age-based reporting recommendation for benign-appearing endometrial cells. Because of the already noted difficulty in identifying atypia in endometrial cells, there has been ongoing controversy over when to report their presence on cervical cytology [2].

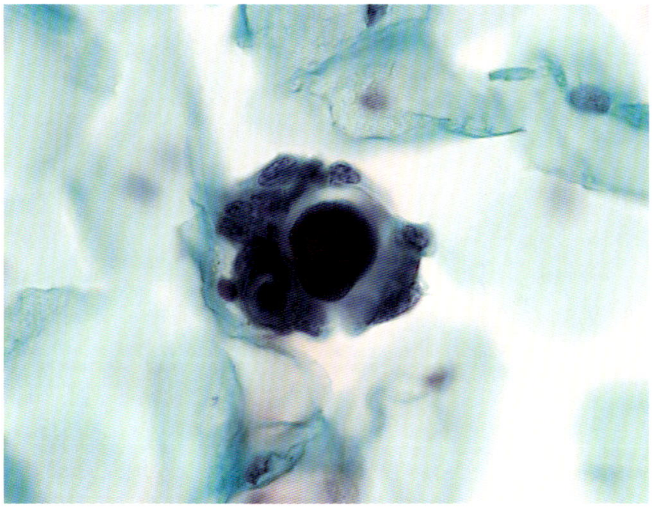

Fig. 2.17. Psammoma bodies. This cluster has a central psammomatous calcification with surrounding malignant cells of serous papillary carcinoma. LBP, SurePath.

Everyone can agree that any endometrial cells encountered in the Pap test of an elderly woman should cause alarm because of the significant risk of underlying malignancy. Some mechanism for reporting such cells is appropriate and important. The difficulty arises in defining an acceptable cutoff point. Regularly menstruating women often shed endometrial cells into Pap tests, even during the second half of the cycle, but rarely develop endometrial adenocarcinoma. Endometrial cells are seen with decreasing frequency in peri- and post-menopausal women as they age, with a corresponding gradual increase in their clinical significance when they do appear. Therefore, there is no tidy and convenient way to determine when benign-appearing endometrial cells are important enough to report. This problem is only compounded by a lack of menstrual history on many Pap test requisitions. The 1991 BS recommended reporting endometrial cells in postmenopausal women as an 'epithelial cell abnormality', but this recommendation was abandoned due to its impracticality [18].

The 2001 BS has established a cutoff point for the reporting of benign-appearing endometrial cells at age 40 regardless of menstrual history. Reporting applies only to exfoliated and intact endometrial cells; abraded lower uterine segment epithelium, stromal cells, and histiocytes are excluded because they do not imply a cancer risk. Vigorous lower uterine segment sampling may result in characteristic large biphasic cell clusters with tubular glands embedded in spindly stroma with blood vessels. Directly sampled histiocytes, and some stromal cells, may appear individually as high nucleus-to-cytoplasm ratio cells with foamy cytoplasm and bean-shaped small nuclei. These patterns are fairly easily recognized in some cases but definitively separating abraded from exfoliated endometrial cells often presents a challenge.

Benign appearing endometrial cells in women over age 40 years should be reported under the interpretive category of 'other', allowing the Pap test to be signed out as 'negative for squamous intraepithelial lesion, endometrials cells over 40' thus alerting the ordering physician to the presence of endometrial cells. An optional comment may also be included. If the endometrial cells are seen in a woman known to be in the first half of her menstrual cycle, the comment may state that the cells correlate with the menstrual history. Otherwise, the comment may state that endometrial cells are usually derived from a benign process, with only a small proportion of women with this finding having endometrial abnormalities. Because these cells are reported as a potential indicator of malignancy, most laboratories choose to send them for pathologist review. However, this is not required by the BS or state/federal regulations in the United States.

2.6. Impact of the 2001 Bethesda System

Some of the important effects of the 1991 BS were an emphasis on criteria for diagnostic categories and descriptors for specimen adequacy for cervical/vaginal cytology. In particular, AGUS became a hot topic with numerous studies investigating its frequency and the results of follow-up biopsies. A recent meta-analysis of this literature found that AGUS accounted for about 0.3% of all Pap test interpretations, with most studies below 1% [14]. The same study, interestingly, found that the most common findings on biopsy follow-up were squamous abnormalities. Less than 10% of AGUS corresponded to true glandular lesions. About 5% were malignant and, disappointingly, more than 70% showed no dysplasia or malignancy on follow-up. AGUS, as a category, was also plagued by concerns about its inter-observer reproducibility [5, 10].

Based on further experience with morphology, follow-up studies and introduction of liquid based gynecologic cytology, the 2001 version of the BS made several changes to the criteria for interpretation and reporting of atypical glandular cells. In an effort to provide guidance for follow-up, specification of site of origin is now encouraged, with accompanying criteria specific for endocervical and endometrial atypia. Unfortunately, recent studies have continued to show poor reproducibility for AGC [1] and its subcategories [16]. Greater success has been demonstrated with respect to indicators of the degree of concern. There is essentially universal agreement that elimination of the subcategory 'favor reactive' has been of benefit by reducing clinical confusion. The addition of the subcategory 'favor neoplastic' may also prove helpful. Studies using this category have found that this subgroup does indeed have a higher incidence of significant lesions found on follow-up [4, 5].

The creation of a separate interpretive category for AIS may likewise improve the clinical usefulness of the 2001 BS by indicating a higher-risk subset of women. When AIS is identified on a Pap test, the follow-up does not always reveal a significant lesion [12]. Most women with AIS discovered in biopsies do not have prior Pap tests interpreted as AIS [7, 15]. This fact may in part be attributable to sampling. However, analysis of the results of cytology surveys show that AIS is much less readily identified than squamous high-grade lesions in Pap tests [11].

Investigations of the utility of reporting benign-appearing endometrial cells in women ≥40 years of age have also been discouraging. Numerous studies have shown that only a very small fraction of such cases correspond to endometrial hyperplasia or malignancy [2]. Furthermore, most of the women with underlying malignancy have symptomatic bleeding, reducing the value of Pap test findings even in true positive cases [3]. After the implementation of the 2001 BS, despite a large increase in the reporting of benign-appearing endometrial cells, the frequency of discovery of EmA has not increased [19].

2.7. Management

In acknowledgement of the significant risk of high-grade lesions/cancer associated with AGC or AIS, the ASCCP guidelines [23] recommend colposcopy and endocervical sampling follow-up for all AGC. Endometrial sampling is also recommended in women ≥35 years of age and in younger women with clinical suspicion of endometrial pathology. For women with negative follow-up of AGC NOS, follow-up with high-risk HPV testing at 12 months is recommended, with a negative HPV result before a return to routine screening. Women with AIS or AGC favor neoplastic, with negative initial work-up, should undergo diagnostic cervical conization. Benign-appearing endometrial cells should prompt endometrial assessment in postmenopausal women and no follow-up in asymptomatic women who are still menstruating.

References

1 Confortini M, Di Bonito L, Carozzi F, Ghiringhello B, Montanari G, Parisio F, Prandi S: Interlaboratory reproducibility of atypical glandular cells of undetermined significance: a national survey. Cytopathology 2006;17:353–360.

2 Fadare O, Ghofrani M, Chacho MS, Parkash V: The significance of benign endometrial cells in cervicovaginal smears. Adv Anat Pathol 2005;12: 274–287.

3 Gomez-Fernandez CR, Ganjei-Azar P, Capote-Dishaw J, Averette HE, Nadji M: Reporting normal endometrial cells in Pap smears: an outcome appraisal. Gynecol Oncol 1999;74:381–384.

4 Chiung-Ru L, Chih-Yi H, Shyh-Haw T, Fen-Yau Lii A: Clinical significance of atypical glandular cells by the 2001 Bethesda System in cytohistologic correlation. Acta Cytol 2008;52:563–567.

5 Yick-Kwong L, Ng WK: Follow-up study of atypical glandular cells in gynecologic cytology using conventional Pap smears and liquid-based preparations: impact of the Bethesda System 2001. Acta Cytol 2008;52:159–168.

6 Lee KR, Darragh TM, Joste NE, Krane JF, Sherman ME, Hurley LB, Allred EM, Manos MM: Atypical glandular cells of undetermined significance (AGUS): Interobserver reproducibility in cervical smears and corresponding thin-layer preparations. Am J Clin Pathol 2002;117:96–102.

7 Mitchell H, Hocking J, Saville M: Cervical cytology screening history of women diagnosed with adenocarcinoma in situ of the cervix: a case-control study. Acta Cytol 2004;48:595–600.

8 Moriarty A.T, Wilbur D: Those gland problems in cervical cytology: faith or fact? Observations from the Bethesda 2001 terminology conference. Diagn Cytopathol 2003;28:171–174.

9 Ozkan F, Ramzy I, Mody DR: Glandular lesions of the cervix on thin-layer Pap tests: validity of cytologic criteria used in identifying significant lesions. Acta Cytol 2004;48:372–379.

10 Raab SS, Geisinger KS, Silverman JF, Thomas PA, Stanley MW: Interobserver variability of a Papanicolaou smear diagnosis of atypical glandular cells of undetermined significance. Am J Clin Pathol 1998;110:653–659.

11 Renshaw AA, Mody DR, Lozano RL, Volk EE, Walsh MK, Davey DD, Birdsong GG: Detection of adenocarcinoma in situ of the cervix in Papanicolaou tests: comparison of diagnostic accuracy with other high-grade lesions. Arch Pathol Lab Med 2004;128:153–157.

12 Roberts JM, Thurloe JK, Biro C, Hyne SG, Williams KE, Bowditch RC: Follow-up of cytologic predictions of endocervical glandular abnormalities: histologic outcomes in 123 cases. J Low Genit Tract Dis 2005;9:71–77.

13 Salomao DR, Hughes GH, Raab SS: Atypical glandular cells of undetermined significance favor endometrial origin: criteria for separating low grade endometrial adenocarcinoma from benign endometrial lesions. Acta Cytol 2002;46:458–464.

14 Schnatz PF, Guile M, O'Sullivan DM, Sorosky JL: Clinical significance of atypical glandular cells on cervical cytology. Obstet Gynecol 2006;107: 701–708.

15 Schoolland M, Segal A, Allpress S, Miranda A, Frost FA, Sterrett OF: Adenocarcinoma in situ of the cervix. Cancer 2002;96:330–337.

16 Simsir A, Hwang S, Cangiarella J, Elgert P, Levine P, Sheffield MV, Roberson J, Talley L, Chhieng DC: Glandular cell atypia on Papanicolaou smears: interobserver variability in the diagnosis and prediction of cell of origin. Cancer 2003;99:323–330.

17 Solomon D, Nayar R: The Bethesda System for Reporting Cervical Cytology: Definitions, Criteria, and Explanatory Notes, ed 2. New York, Springer, 2004.

18 Solomon D, Davey D, Kurman R, Moriarty A, O'Connor D, Prey M, Raab S, Sherman M, Wilbur D, Wright T, Young N: The 2001 Bethesda System: terminology for reporting results of cervical cytology. JAMA 2002;287:2114–2119.

19 Thrall, M, Kjeldahl K, Savik K, Gulbahce HE, Pambuccian SE: Rate of endometrial adenocarcinoma in women screened before and after implementation of the Bethesda 2001 reporting system. Acta Cytol 2008;52:1–7.

20 van Aspert-van Erp AJ, Smedts FM, Vooijs GP: Severe cervical glandular cell lesions and severe cervical combined lesions: predictive value of the Papanicolaou smear. Cancer 2004;102:210–207.

21 Wang SS, Sherman ME, Hildesheim A, Lacey JV, Devesa S: Cervical adenocarcinoma and squamous cell carcinoma incidence trends among white women and black women in the United States for 1976–2000. Cancer 2004;100:1035–1044.

22 Wood MD, Horst JA, Bibbo M: Weeding atypical glandular cell look-alikes from the true atypical lesions in liquid-based Pap tests: a review. Diagn Cytopathol 2007;35:12–17.

23 Wright TC, Massad LS, Dunton JC, Spitzer M, Wilkinson EJ, Solomon D: 2006 Consensus guidelines for the management of women with abnormal cervical cancer screening tests. Am J Obstet Gynecol 2007;197:346–355.

Chapter 3

Cytopathology of the Benign Glandular Lesions of the Cervix and Glandular Cytopathology of the Vagina

3.1. Cytopathology of Benign Glandular Lesions of the Cervix

3.1.1. Benign tumors

3.1.1.1. Endocervical Polyp

Considered by some as a neoplasm, by others as hyperplasia, the endocervical polyp (EP) is a very common lesion, especially in multi-gravidae, and rare before menarche. It is usually asymptomatic but may occasionally cause intermittent or post-coital bleeding. It appears as a lobulated, polypoid growth projecting from the endocervical os. It is benign with no malignant potential, but cancer can occasionally arise in an EP. Most endocervical polyps are discovered during gynaecological examination.

Histologically, an EP is composed of a central connective tissue stalk lined by endocervical, squamous or metaplastic squamous epithelium. The stroma contains blood vessels and endocervical glands.

EP has no specific cytological pattern, except for the rare finding of a fragment of a polyp in smears (fig. 3.1). Such tissue fragments have smooth borders lined by columnar cells, pale intermediate zones and dark inner cores of numerous small, dark stromal cells [34]. Otherwise, smears present considerable numbers of benign endocervical cells, shedding in large sheets or forming glands, and presence of metaplastic cells.

Berzolla et al. describe reactive atypia in 1.6%, inflammatory changes in 27.7%, metaplasia in 13.6% and microgladular hyperplasia in 6.8% of the 2,246 EP they studied. Sampling of theses processes can lead to a cytological diagnosis of 'presence of atypical endocervical cells' or even to a false positive diagnosis of adenocarcinoma. On the other hand, EP showed dysplasia in 0.5% of cases and malignancy was diagnosed in 0.1%, although none of the cases were primary [7]. Jiménez-Ayala described a case of a serous surface papillary carcinoma of the ovary metastatic to an EP. The diagnosis of adenocarcinoma was made in a routine cervicovaginal smear, and the primitive tumor was later found in an ovary (fig. 3.2) [23].

Another cytological problem is the frequency of unsatisfactory Pap smears. The presence of EP is one of the commonest causes of unsatisfactory specimens, with vaginal bleeding and postpartum status [25].

3.1.1.2. Müllerian Papilloma

Müllerian papilloma is a rare benign tumor of the cervix and/or vagina that occurs predominantly in young children. The cytological findings in a benign Müllerian papilloma

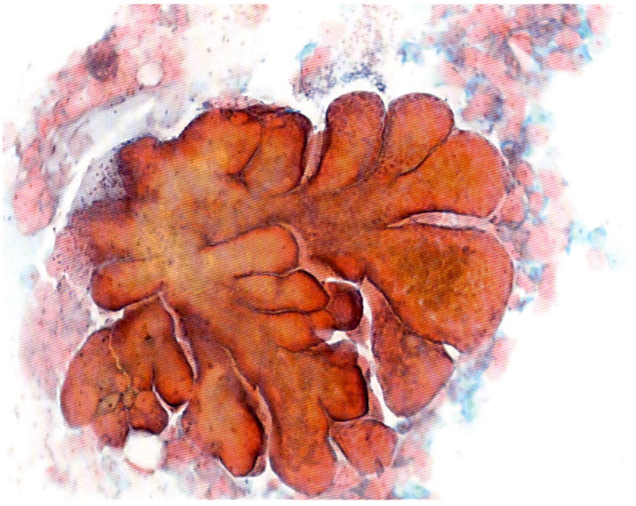

Fig. 3.1. Cytological features of an endocervical polyp are unspecific, except when a fragment of polyp is present in the smear.

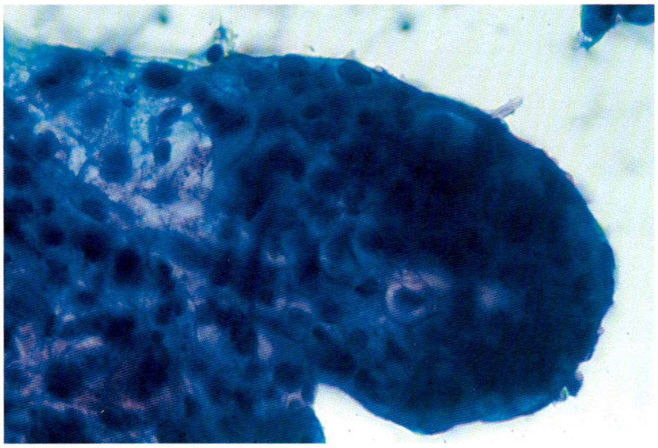

Fig. 3.2. A carcinoma of the ovary metastatic to an endocervical polyp was suspected in a routine cervicovaginal smear.

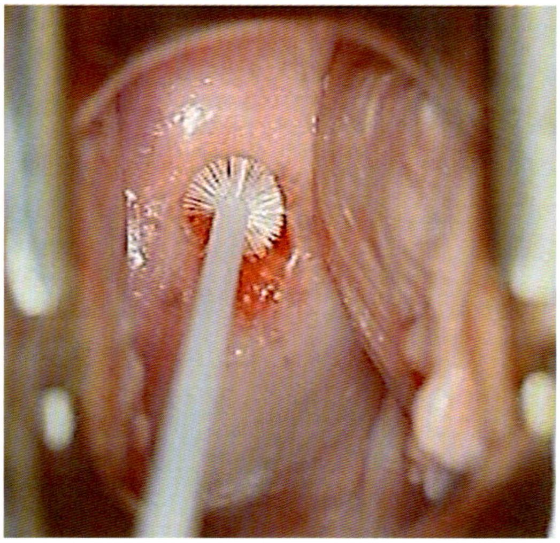

Fig. 3.3. The extensive use of endocervical brush instruments has increase the number of cases reported as AGC.

have been described only in 1 report [22]. The cytology seen in touch preparation, ThinPrep, and cell block preparations from a 15-month-old girl was of a cellular specimen containing complex papillary fronds composed of overlapping and crowded small hyperchromatic cells with a high nuclear:cytoplasmic ratio, and feathering that resembled a malignant neoplasm.

3.1.2. Other Non-Tumoral Lesions

Endocervical brush instruments are now widely used to secure cells from the endocervical canal and assure adequacy of sampling (fig. 3.3). This has resulted in an increasing rate of detection and increasing attention to glandular abnormalities of the cervix. The number of 'Satisfactory for evaluation but limited by the absence of endocervical/transformation component' smears has decreased, but there has also been a rise in the number of cases reported as presence of 'atypical glandular cells' (AGC). An AGC diagnosis is often of more concern than a diagnosis of 'atypical squamous cells of undetermined significance' (ASC-US), since most patients with an AGC diagnosis have a significant cervicalw lesion, most commonly a high-grade squamous intraepithelial lesion. Other clinically important diagnoses of AGC in histology are endocervical adenocarcinoma in situ (AIS), squamous intraepithelial lesion (SIL) extending into a glandular space and endocervical adenocarcinoma.

3.1.2.1. Tubal Metaplasia

Tubal metaplasia (TM) is a benign, non-neoplastic replacement of the normal endocervical (or endometrial) epithelium with cells characteristic of the fallopian tube: ciliated clear cells, non-ciliated secretory cells, and intercalated (or peg) cells. TM is very common. Babkowski et al. demonstrated its presence in all of the 25 hysterectomy specimens with no history of cervical disease they studied. TM was more prominent in the upper third of the endocervical canal [4]. With the increased use of endocervical sampling devices, this site of the canal is more frequently sampled, and TM is now a fairly common finding in cervicovaginal smear (CVS). There is a general agreement that TM is not a lesion with malignant potential, but rather a probable hormone-induced change, without neoplastic progression. However, Schlesinger and Silverberg state that it cannot be assumed that all ciliated tubal epithelium in the cervix is benign with no premalignant potential. For theses authors, the relationship of atypical TM (dysplasia) to tubal-type AIS should be defined, and this pattern should be added to the known types of differentiation of cervical AIS, such as endocervical, endometrioid or intestinal [44].

TM presents as flat sheets or cohesive 3-dimensional aggregates with regular nuclear spacing. The cells are columnar, with apical terminal bars with cilia. Nuclei are regular, oval to elongate, and typically polarized to the basal portions of the cells. Chromatin is finely to moderately granular with small or inconspicuous nucleoli. Mitoses are rare and the background is clean. Most of these cytologic features are best observed when cells are in a palisading arrangement. The diagnosis of

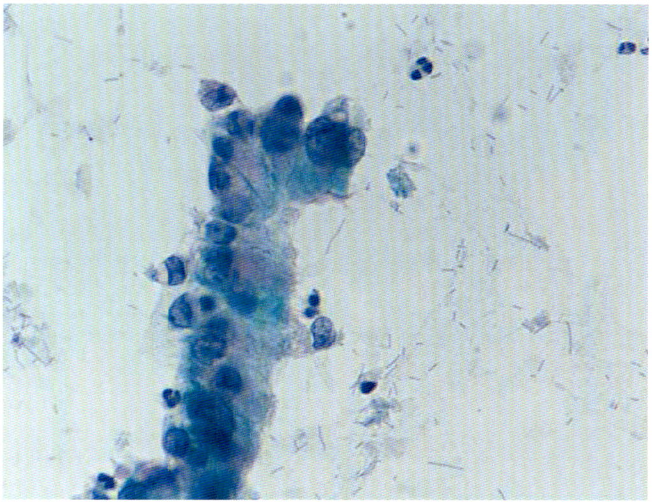

Fig. 3.4. The diagnosis of tubal metaplasia becomes obvious when cilia are well seen and are prominently present.

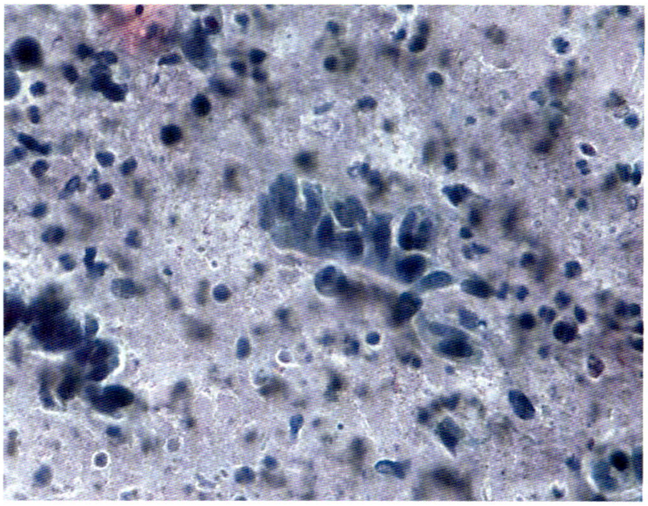

Fig. 3.5. AIS is the most important differential diagnosis of tubal metaplasia. Cilia are absent and nuclei are larger, more crowded with elongation, anisonucleosis, and coarse granularity.

TM becomes obvious when cilia are well seen and are prominently present (fig. 3.4). However, cilia are particularly susceptible to drying artifacts, and a diagnosis of TM and its distinction from other glandular lesions may not be possible.

The distinction of AIS from TM is a major problem (fig. 3.5) [14, 35]. Novotny el al. found that TM accounted for 76% of the abnormalities in which cervical cytology suggested a possible diagnosis of preinvasive glandular neoplasia [35]. AIS generally shows moderate to high cellularity, numerous crowded sheets, feathered edges easily seen in isolated strips, and rosette formations. Terminal bars and cilia are absent, while nuclei are larger, more crowded and palisaded, and characterized by elongation, anisonucleosis, and coarse granularity. Mitoses are usually seen.

Endometriosis and atypical inflammatory or reactive changes should also be included in the differential diagnosis. Some ciliated cells can also be seen in normal endocervical epithelium, although they are a minority of the total endocervical exfoliation, and their nuclei do not show enlargement or even moderate anisonucleosis as possibly seen in TM.

3.1.2.2. Microglandular Hyperplasia

Microglandular hyperplasia (MGH), first described by Taylor and Norris in 1967, is characterized by a benign proliferation of endocervical glands (fig. 3.6). This lesion was classically found in young women and was associated with pregnancy and contraceptive use. However, MGH has also been observed in postmenopausal women [1], in the absence of contraceptive medication, and in some cases, without any obvious cause. MGH is usually an incidental finding, but may cause a gross abnormality, most commonly a polyp. In histology, MGH consists of closely packed irregular glands, lined by benign endocervical cells.

Some reports have tried to define specific cytomorphologic features. Alvarez-Santin described for the first time cytomorphologic criteria for the diagnosis of MGH. Typical cell clusters showing microlumina or fenestrated spaces with shared walls and an admixture of glandular cells, immature squamous metaplastic and subcylindrical reserve cells give the clue to the diagnosis (fig. 3.7) [1]. Shidham et al. describe 2 possible patterns: a glandular pattern characterized by mucin-depleted endocervical cells in 3-dimensional groups with microlumina and a metaplastic pattern consisting of groups of immature squamous metaplastic cells usually as a checkerboard-like arrangement or as streaks of single metaplastic cells in a row. This metaplastic pattern can lead to interpretations of 'atypical squamous cells – high grade SIL not excluded' (ASC-H) [48]. DeMay describes pseudoparakeratosis as a possible clue to MGH [11]. Pseudoparakeratosis was described by Patten in 1978 [37] and is characterized by numerous single, degenerated endocervical cells, often in linear arrays in conventional smears, that typically have pyknotic nuclei and orangeophilic cytoplasm.

Many cytological features of MGH in CVS have been described, although they appear to be nonspecific. Much of the emphasis in the literature on this entity has been on the

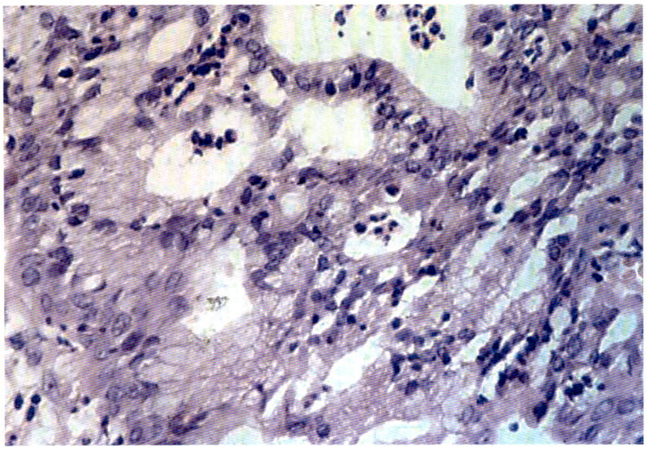

Fig. 3.6. Microglandular hyperplasia is a benign proliferation of endocervical glands. Image courtesy of Dr. Alvarez-Santín.

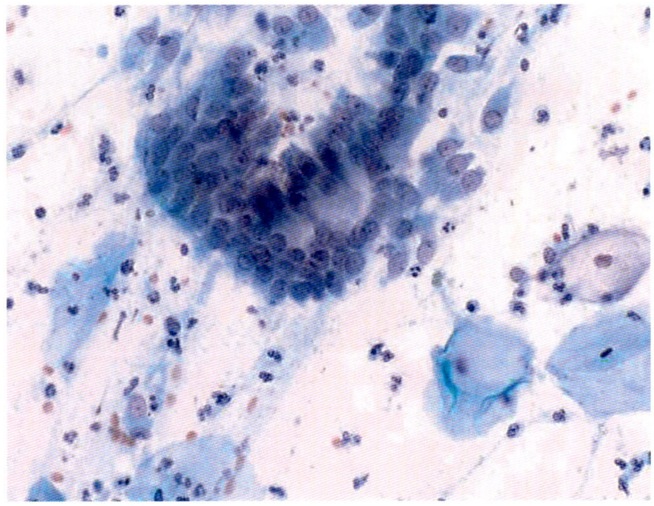

Fig. 3.7. Microglandular hyperplasia showing cell clusters with microlumina and an admixture of glandular cells, immature squamous metaplastic and subcylindrical reserve cells. Image courtesy of Dr. Alvarez-Santín.

features that enable the pathologist to avoid misinterpreting this benign process as adenocarcinoma or SIL. In fact, rare atypical forms of MGH have been described [59] in which nuclear enlargement, hyperchromasia, coarsening of the chromatin, nuclear crowding and cellular overlap were seen in smears [2, 52]. Absence of irregular nuclear membranes, and 'feathery' edges or presence of cells with cilia or terminal bars point to a benign interpretation [52].

3.1.2.3. Cells of the Lower Uterine Segment

The lower uterine segment (LUS), also called the 'isthmus of the cervix', is an anatomical region, largely endometrial but partly transitional from the endocervix, that is less responsive to hormone stimulation than the endometrium of the uterine corpus. Its epithelium, stroma and vasculature recapitulate the functional state of inactive endometrium. In tissue sections the LUS has short, poorly developed, inactive glands that are dispersed in a stroma consisting of elongated fibroblast-like cells.

The routine use of endocervical brushes has made the transition zone between cervix and endometrium more accessible to sampling. The presence of LUS cells in CVS of patients who have undergone cervical cone biopsy has also been reported [24]. In a prospective study, De Peralta-Venturino et al. showed cells of the LUS in 0.55% of a total of 62,187 smears studied [12].

Endometrial cells present in the second half of the menstrual cycle or abnormally present in the post-menopause generally consist of small cell balls, which may or may not be surrounded by packed stromal cells. Endometrial cells of the LUS do not shed 'spontaneously', but are abraded as large tissue fragments in brush collections, like direct endometrial sampling.

The cells of the LUS obtained by endocervical brushings present as large tissue fragments of endometrial stroma with and without tubular glands, often with a branching pattern. Gland openings are often visible. The admixture of glandular and stromal components is best seen at low-power magnification. The glandular cells contain round nuclei with finely granular chromatin. Extreme nuclear crowding with occasional peripheral palisading is sometimes seen and mitoses are easily found. The stromal cells are uniform, round to spindle shaped with oval nuclei, have a finely granular chromatin and scant cytoplasm. Capillaries traversing the stromal tissue fragments are characteristic (fig. 3.8) [12].

LUS cells may be mistaken for normal cells or cells of benign processes such as endocervical tissue, sheets of parabasal cells in atrophic smears, endometrial cells shed in women with an intrauterine device, exogenous hormones or endometrial pathology, endometriosis or tubal metaplasia. More attention has to be given to the differential diagnosis of LUS cells with neoplastic lesions such as endocervical carcinoma in situ, squamous carcinoma in situ and well differentiated endometrial adenocarcinoma.

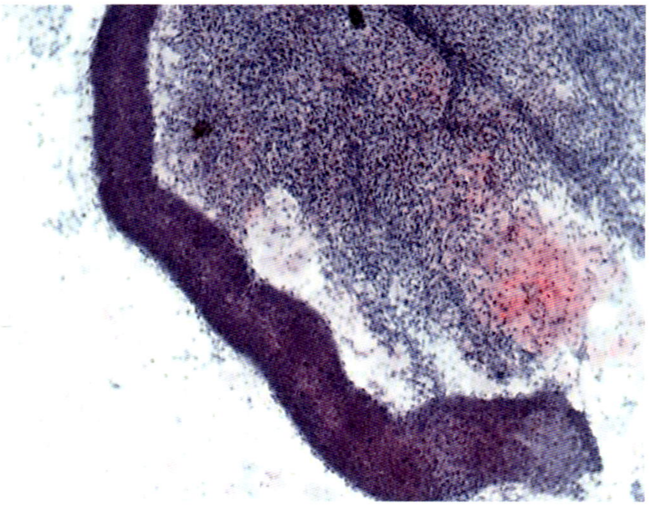

Fig. 3.8. Tubular glands with capillaries traversing large tissue fragments of endometrial stroma are characteristic of cells of the lower uterine segment.

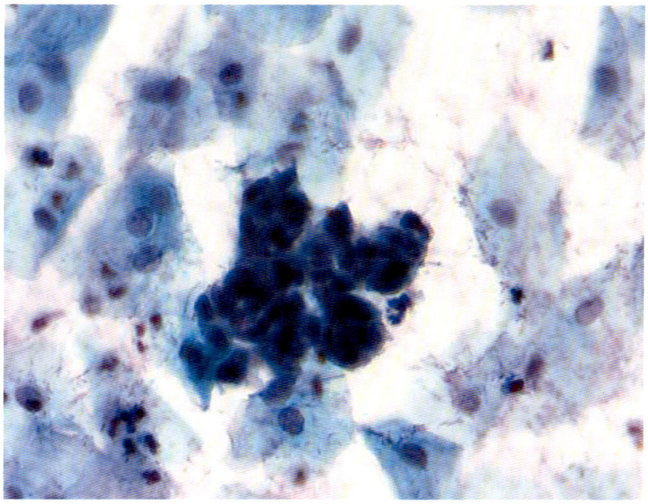

Fig. 3.9. Specific recognition of cervical endometriosis is usually not possible in cervicovaginal smears. Only hyperchromatic crowded groups of endometrial epithelial cells are usually seen.

3.1.2.4. Endometriosis

Endometriosis is the presence of endometrial type tissue outside the endometrium. Regarded as infrequent, cervical endometriosis (CE) probably occurs more commonly than is generally realized. Clinically, endometriosis can be asymptomatic or present with unspecific symptoms such as persistent post-coital or intermenstrual bleeding. Areas of CE appear as 1 or more small blue or red surface nodules, and are more frequent following trauma, such as biopsy or delivery. Colposcopy and cervical biopsy are basic techniques to make the diagnosis. Fine needle aspiration cytology has been applied to the diagnosis of cervical endometriosis [53].

There are 2 types of CE: deep CE (which is usually associated with pelvic endometriosis) and superficial CE. When the glands are rare or absent in superficial CE, the term stromal endometriosis is used [10]. Because of its location, superficial CE may be sampled by current endocervical sampling devices. The classic triad for endometriosis is the presence of endometrial glandular cells, endometrial sromal cells and hemosiderin-laden macrophages, but the full triad is generally not present in smears. Smears are usually bloody with degenerated red blood cells and presence of strips, sheets and hyperchromatic crowded groups of endometrial epithelial cells (fig. 3.9). Specific recognition of cervical endometriosis is usually not possible in CVS and the importance of CE is that it can simulate malignancy. Glandular groups may show nuclear crowding, pseudostratification, focal 'feathering' and rare rosettes. The cells may show nuclear hyperchromasia or pleomorphism, and nucleoli may or may not be visible [18, 27, 32, 50]. CE shows variable features in cytological specimens, partly due to the menstrual cycle hormonal changes which are similar in endometriotic tissue and functioning endometrium [27]. Recognition of endometrial stroma in continuity with groups of cells with these features on CVS may suggest the diagnosis of CE [50]. However, there is sufficient overlap with the cytological features of precancerous and cancerous glandular lesions for most cases of CE to be diagnosed as AGC.

3.1.2.5. Arias-Stella Reaction

In 1954, Arias-Stella described for the first time the presence of marked nuclear atypism in hypersecretory endometrial glands during pregnancy. Similar abnormalities may be observed in histologic sections of the endocervical epithelium. Schneider observed the endocervical Arias-Stella reaction (ASR) in 9% of hysterectomy specimens obtained during pregnancy [45]. Similar changes may also be observed in the endometrial and endocervical epithelium of women on hormonal therapy, receiving contraceptive hormones with high progesterone content, with oral progestational agents for the management of dysfunctional uterine bleeding or undergoing infertility treatment [13, 26].

ASR of the endocervix has a varied histologic appearance and can show intraglandular tufts, delicate filiform papillae or cribriform intraglandular growth. Cells show marked atypia and have an oxyphilic or vacuolated clear cytoplasm and frequent presence of intranuclear pseudoinclusions. Hobnail cells and occasional mitosis can also be present (fig. 3.10) [36].

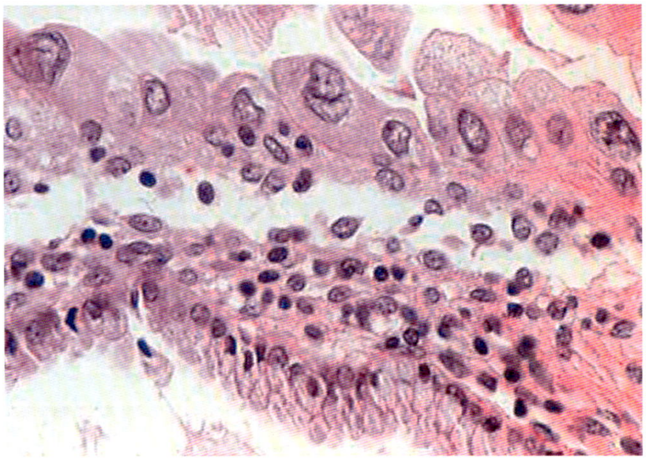

Fig. 3.10. Arias-Stella reaction may be observed in endometrial and also in endocervical epithelium. Image courtesy of Dr. Schneider.

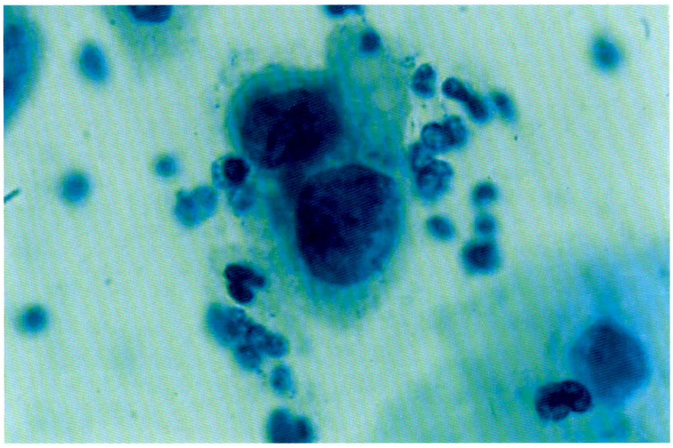

Fig. 3.11. Arias-Stella reaction is characterized by cells with a large, atypical nucleus and abundant, clear or vacuolated cytoplasm. Image courtesy of Dr. Schneider.

Glandular changes encountered in cytological material are similar to those described in histology. ASR is characterized by large cells with a single, large, round to oval nucleus with smudgy chromatin imparting a ground glass appearance, frequent intranuclear inclusions and vacuolated to dense, variable cytoplasm (fig. 3.11) [6]. The changes involving endocervical glandular epithelium are often alarming and the cytologic diagnoses usually range from 'presence of AGC' to a false positive diagnosis of adenocarcinoma, mainly of clear cell type. The significance of such cell changes as a potential diagnostic pitfall in cytology has largely been emphasized. The clinical history is of critical diagnostic value in the assessment of such cells that otherwise may readily be mistaken for cancer cells. On the other hand, not only benign changes such as ASR are found in CVS of pregnant and postpartum women. Several studies show the existence of low- and high-grade squamous intraepithelial lesions in an important number of cases, sometimes confirmed after a cytological diagnosis of AGC in the CVS [9, 29, 38].

3.2. Glandular Cytopathology of the Vagina

3.2.1. Tumoral Lesions

3.2.1.1. Benign Tumoral Lesions: Adenomas

The adenomas of the vagina are benign glandular tumors with enteric differentiation, probably arising from cloacal remnants. The adenomas are histologically similar to colonic types and have been subclassified as tubular, tubulovillous or villous. Adenocarcinoma arising from a vaginal adenoma has been reported [31].

The most important lesions in the differential diagnosis are metastatic carcinoma to the vagina and extension or recurrence of endometrial or endocervical adenocarcinoma.

Vaginal adenomas are extremely rare and no cytological descriptions have been reported.

3.2.1.2. Malignant Tumoral Lesions: Adenocarcinomas

3.2.1.2.1. Clear Cell Adenocarcinoma

Adenocarcinomas of the vagina are rare, although they assumed more importance in the generation of women afflicted with diethylstilbestrol (DES)-induced vaginal adenosis (AD). DES was prescribed for threatened or repeated miscarriage from the 1941 to the early 1970s. Millions of women were exposed in utero to this and related drugs in several countries, including the Unites States, France and the Netherlands. There was an increase in incidence of clear cell adenocarcinoma (CCA) in young women, mainly between 14 and 22 years in the 1970s, and then a second smaller peak at age 70 years was found. In fact, a bimodal age distribution has also been recorded in cases without intrauterine DES exposure. The risk for CCA to develop in an exposed female from birth to age 34 has been estimated to be 1 case per 1,000 women [28]. The rarity of this tumor among exposed women suggests that DES is not a complete carcinogen. A carcinogenesis-promoting role of menarche and menopause and/or the existence of a subpopulation with genetic or exogenous risk factors other than exposure to DES have been suggested [19].

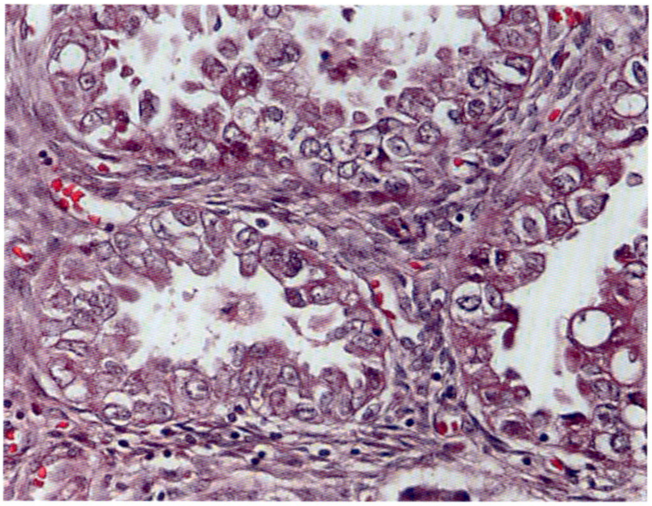

Fig. 3.12. Clear cell adenocarcinoma of the vagina has an appearance similar to those arising in the cervix, endometrium and ovary.

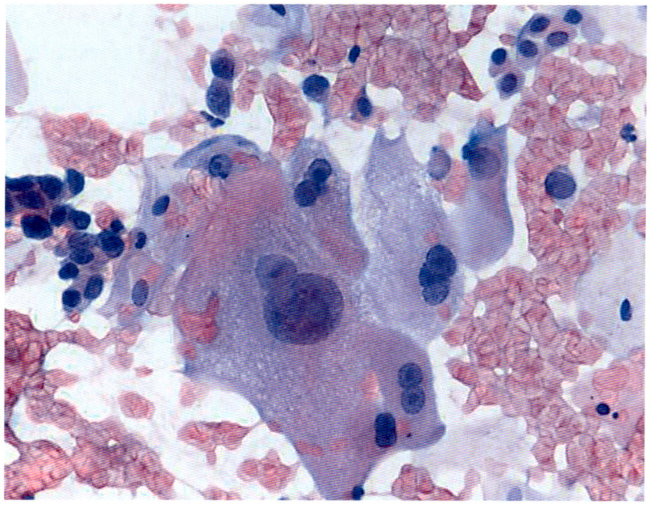

Fig. 3.13. Clear cell adenocarcinoma present cells with abundant, transparent, sometimes vacuolated cytoplasm and large nuclei with prominent nucleoli.

Whilst any part of the vagina may be involved, CCA most often arises from its upper part. On the other hand, vaginal metastases of renal carcinoma generally occur in the lower third of the vagina and this information can be important in the differential diagnosis. A primary vaginal CCA may also involve the cervix. According to the FIGO criteria about two thirds of CCA following DES exposure are classified as tumors of the vagina and one third of the cervix [19]. In non-DES-exposed young women and post-menopausal women this ratio is reversed. CCA has been described in women with vaginal endometriosis [47].

Vaginal bleeding, discharge and dyspareunia are the most common symptoms, but women may be asymptomatic. CCA typically are polypoid, nodular, or papillary but may also be flat or ulcerated. Histologicaly, CCA of the vagina has an appearance similar to those arising in the cervix, endometrium and ovary. The most common pattern is tubulocystic, but it also may be solid or mixed. The cells have a characteristic clear cytoplasm that gives the tumor its name. Hobnail cells are also present, characterized by inconspicuous cytoplasm and a bulbous nucleus that protrudes into the glandular lumen (fig. 3.12).

Cytological examination can detect adenocarcinoma and also serves as a follow-up procedure after treatment of the lesion. If the uterine cervix is involved, the cervical scrape smear is very efficient at detecting the tumor. If only the vagina is involved, the cervical smear fails to reveal the tumor in many cases. Thus, a vaginal pool smear in young women, particularly those at risk for AD and adenocarcinoma, is important. The cells in vaginal CCA are present singly or in sheets, clusters, or occasionally papillae. The cytoplasm is abundant, delicate and transparent, sometimes with small vacuoles. The nuclei are large, round to irregular with prominent nucleoli (fig. 3.13). Naked nuclei are common owing to the delicate nature of the cytoplasm. If the tumor is ulcerated, evidence of inflammation and necrosis is usually present. If there is adjacent residual AD, in the vagina or in the cervix, benign cells of endocervical type may be present and may confuse the cytological picture.

CCA is generally well recognized on cytology when tumoral cells are present in the smears. But a vaginal origin should not be established before ruling out an origin in the cervix, endometrium or ovary, or a metastasis from the urinary tract (see chapter 11). The diagnosis of primary CCA of the vagina should be made based on a normal cytopathologic examination of the cervix, endometrium and ascites, normal appearance of the uterus, ovaries and kidneys on MRI, and absence of detectable tumor in the urinary tract [54].

3.2.1.2.2. Endometrioid Adenocarcinoma

Although it is probably the second most frequent primary adenocarcinoma of the vagina, only a few primary endometriod adenocarcinomas of the vagina have been reported, most of them arising in vaginal endometriosis. The largest series included 18 cases [49].The patients ranged from 45 to 81 years of age. Most presented with vaginal bleeding, and had had a prior hysterectomy. Five had a history of unopposed estrogen therapy but none had a history of intrauterine DES exposure. Vaginal endometriosis was identified in 14 cases, and is an important indication of a primary vaginal tumor, rather than secondary spread from the endometrium.

The histological and cytological appearance resembles that of the much more common endometrioid adenocarcinoma of the endometrium. The cytological features depend mainly on the level of differentiation, with larger, and more pleomorphic and atypical cells in high-grade tumors. Generally, the tumor sheds loose clusters of relatively small cells (syncytial balls), with eccentric, round nuclei, fine to coarse chromatin, small nucleoli and scant cytolplasm. Other subtypes of adenocarcinoma (such as serous when the tumor has a papillary pattern) and atypical forms of endometriosis, are the most common differential diagnostic considerations.

3.2.1.2.3. Mucinous Adenocarcinoma

Primary mucinous adenocarcinoma (MA) of the vagina is rare, with few cases reported. Two MA have been described in neovaginas, formed to correct congenital anomalies [21], one of which developed a chronic rectovaginal fistula [33]. Two other MA have been described arising in rectovaginal fistulas associated with Chrohn's disease [30]. It is thought that the MA developed as a result of chronic inflammation secondary to the fistula. Primary MA has also been described associated with adenosis and without history of DES exposure, suggesting a Müllerian origin [55, 58]. The main point may be to differentiate the tumor from a metastatic adenocarcinoma, especially of cervical origin. Sulfomucin has not been found to be different in primary MA vagina cells from most MA cells of the endocervical type [43].

The histological appearance resembles that of the much more common endocervical or intestinal adenocarcinomas of the cervix. Although the few cases reported do not describe the cytological aspects, columnar cells with possible mucous in the cytoplasm and palisading or rosette arrangement would be expected.

3.2.1.2.4. Mesonephric Adenocarcinoma

Mesonephric adenocarcinoma deriving from remnants of vaginal mesonephric (Gartner) ducts is one of the rarest tumors of the female genital tract with very few cases reported, and none of them with cytological description [5, 8, 15]. These tumors are composed of well-formed tubules lined by atypical, mitotically-active, cuboidal to columnar epithelium, generally in a background of mesonephric remnants.

Mesonephric carcinoma is the old designation for the clear cell adenocarcinoma. Unlike this tumor, mesonephric carcinoma does not contain clear or hobnail cells, intracellular mucin or glycogen, and the tubules are often surrounded by a basement membrane.

3.2.2. Non-Tumoral Lesions

3.2.2.1. Adenosis

Adenosis (AD) is the replacement of vaginal squamous epithelium by glandular epithelium. Although there has been considerable speculation as to the pathogenesis of AD, currently it is thought to be the result of the persistence of embryonic Müllerian epithelium.

As explained before, DES was extensively used during the late 1940s and early 1950s, until in 1971 the US Food and Drug Administration advised physicians to stop prescribing DES during pregnancy. AD has been reported to occur in approximately 30% of women after in utero exposure to DES and in up to 8% of unexposed women. Roboy et al. reported 41 patients with this disorder who had no DES exposure [42]. AD of the vagina has also been described after intravaginal application of 5-fluorouracil [17], laser vaporization [46], usually for extensive condylomas of the vulva and vagina, and in a patient on tamoxifen therapy [16].

AD is usually asymptomatic, although some women present with a mucous discharge, bleeding or dyspareunia. AD may spontaneously regress at the surface and the glandular epithelium undergoes squamous metaplasia, which becomes mature and identical to normal squamous epithelium. Thus, unless there is evidence or suspicion of malignant transformation, it appears safe to observe these patients without treatment. The risk that CCA will develop in an exposed female from birth to age 34 has been estimated as 1 case per 1,000 women [28]. Because of the risk of development of CCA within the vaginal wall, palpation, colposcopic examination and cytological smears are necessary to monitor patients with AD.

On colposcopy, AD may be occult or may present as cysts or as a diffusely red granular area, most frequently in the anterior upper third of the vagina and adjacent to the cervix.

AD is characterized by the presence in the vagina of columnar epithelium of the endocervix (mucinous type) or less frequently the endometrium or the fallopian tube (tuboendometrial type) or a mixture of both. AD may be found on the surface or deeper in the stroma. Mixtures of

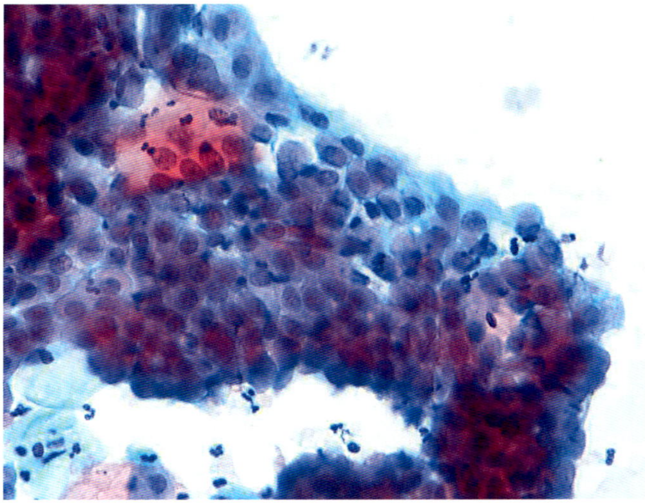

Fig. 3.14. Vaginal adenosis shows glandular cells of endocervical type or squamous metaplasia. Because this is a normal finding in a cervicovaginal smear but not in the vagina, a direct sampling of the lesions is recommended.

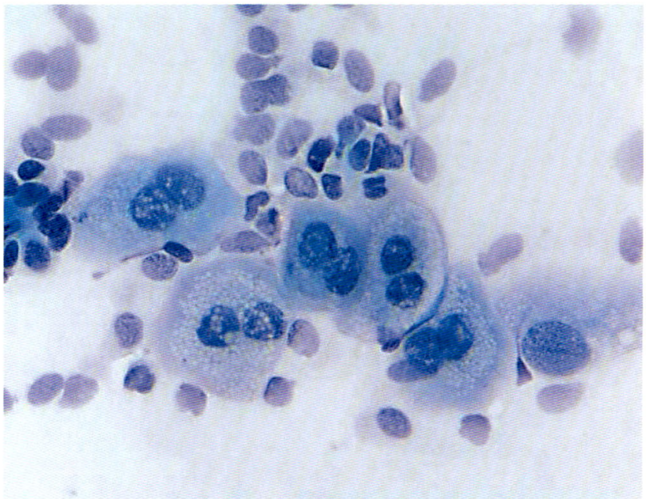

Fig. 3.15. The presence of urothelial cells in a vaginal smear may indicate the existence of a vesicovaginal fistula.

the various types of AD may be encountered. All changes commonly observed in the endocervical epithelium may be observed in AD: tubal metaplasia, squamous metaplasia, and malignant transformation leading to adenocarcinoma, epidemoid carcinoma and its precursor lesions.

Cytology can be helpful in the diagnostic evaluation of DES-exposed women. It may serve a dual purpose, as a means for detection of adenocarcinoma or as a follow-up procedure after treatment of the lesion. The smears show glandular cells of endocervical type or glandular cells showing transition to squamous metaplasia (fig. 3.14). Because this is a normal finding in a CVS, with presence of cells of the transition zone, but not in the vagina, a direct sampling of the lesions, especially under visual control is recommended. AD can be difficult to diagnose, because the glandular epithelium does not desquamate easily and the cytological aspects are not specific [40].

An atypical form of AD has been described and has been reported to be the precursor lesion of CCA [41]. Atypical AD occurs in the tubuloendometrial type of AD and is a frequent finding immediately adjacent to CCA. The atypical glands tend to be more complex than those of mucinous AD and are lined by cells with enlarged, atypical, pleomorphic, hyperchromatic nuclei that contain prominent nucleoli. These atypical glandular cells can be seen in cytology. Squamous dysplasia can also be found. Robboy et al. found high grade intraepithelial lesions or atypical glandular cells in 1% of the 575 women exposed to DES they studied [40].

3.2.2.2. Fistulous Tracts

Fistulous tracts between the vagina and an adjacent organ, such as the rectum (rectovaginal fistula, RVF) or the bladder (vesicovaginal fistula), may result in the presence of epithelial cells of urothelial (fig. 3.15) or intestinal origin in vaginal smears.

Angeles and Saigo studied 23 vaginal smears from women with RVF for different surgical complications. Sixty-five percent of the cases had rectal glandular cells and the diagnosis of a RVF could bemade. Fecal material was found in 30% of the cases. This is suggestive but not diagnostic of RVF [3]. Indigested muscle or vegetable fibers can sometimes be identified. Although malignant glandular cells can be seen in those RVF that arise from direct extension of a colorectal adenocarcinoma, most glandular cells are benign. Columnar, mucus-producing glandular cells generally form compact sheets or clusters with basal nuclei and smooth luminal epithelial surface. The cells need to be distinguished from cells of vaginal adenosis and from endocervical or endometrial benign or malignant cells.

3.2.2.3. Tubal Prolapse

Prolapsed fallopian tube after hysterectomy is a rare but well known complication that has rarely been described in cytological reports. The cells are columnar and occasionally ciliated, with granular nuclei and prominent nucleoli [20, 57]. The cytological findings may help the clinician to

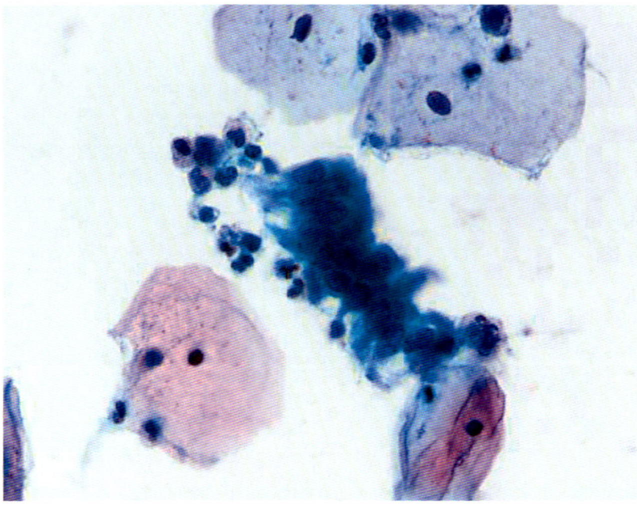

Fig. 3.16. The presence of columnar, ciliated cells in a vaginal smear may indicate a prolapsed fallopian tube after hysterectomy.

differentiate the unusual condition of a prolapsed fallopian tube from other vault 'granulations' (fig. 3.16).

3.2.2.4. Post-Hysterectomy Glandular Cells

Glandular cells in post-hysterectomy women can be seen in different situations, as described in this chapter. Some patients whose smears are received in the laboratory as 'vaginal cuff', have in fact the cervix preserved, and probably a subtotal hysterectomy was then performed. All these causes should been ruled out based on clinical history, colposcopic examination or even biopsy, before reporting post-hysterectomy glandular cells. The origin of these cells is not clear but most authors postulate a possible regenerative response to injury or therapy [39, 51].

The smears show benign glandular cells of endocervical type that cannot be differentiated from those sampled from the endocervix. Three cell types have been described: squamous metaplastic cells, hybrid cells and columnar cells [51]. Based on cytomorphologic criteria alone, benign glandular cells were found in 3.5% of post-hysterectomy vaginal liquid-based Pap tests examined by Ramdall et al. When immunohistochemical (Cytokeratin 7) and special stains (mucicarmine and alcian blue-periodic acid-Schiff) were applied, the percentage of true glandular cells decreased to 1.2% [39].

Post-hysterectomy glandular cells are included in the 2001 Bethesda System in the category 'Other non-neoplastic findings', although reporting them is optional. The presence of these benign cells has little clinical impact, and no special management is recommended.

References

1 Alvarez-Santín C, Sica A, Rodríguez M, Feijó A, Garrido G: Microglandular hyperplasia of the uterine cervix: cytologic diagnosis in cervical smears. Acta Cytol 1999;43:110–113.
2 Alvarez-Santin C: Microglandular hyperplasia of the uterine cervix: cytologic diagnosis in cervical smears. Acta Cytol 2000;44:480–481.
3 Angeles MA, Saigo PE: Cytologic findings in rectovaginal fistulae. Acta Cytol 1994;38:373–376.
4 Babkowski RC, Wilbur DC, Rutkowski MA, Facik MS, Bonfiglio TA: The effects of endocervical canal topography, tubal metaplasia, and high canal sampling on the cytologic presentation of nonneoplastic endocervical cells. Am J Clin Pathol 1996;105:403–410.
5 Bagué S, Rodríguez IM, Prat J: Malignant mesonephric tumors of the female genital tract: a clinicopathologic study of 9 cases. Am J Surg Pathol 2004;28:601–607.
6 Benoit JL, Kini SR: 'Arias-Stella reaction'-like changes in endocervical glandular epithelium in cervical smears during pregnancy and postpartum states: a potential diagnostic pitfall. Diagn Cytopathol 1996;14:349–355.
7 Berzolla CE, Schnatz PF, O'Sullivan DM, Bansal R, Mandavilli S, Sorosky JI: Dysplasia and malignancy in endocervical polyps. J Womens Health (Larchmt) 2007;16:1317–1321.
8 Bifulco G, Mandato VD, Mignogna C, Giampaolino P, Di Spiezio Sardo A, De Cecio R, De Rosa G, Piccoli R, Radice L, Nappi C: A case of mesonephric adenocarcinoma of the vagina with a 1-year follow-up. Int J Gynecol Cancer 2008;18:1127–1131.
9 Chhieng DC, Elgert P, Cangiarella JF, Cohen JM: Significance of AGUS Pap smears in pregnant and postpartum women. Acta Cytol 2001;45:294–299.
10 Clement PB, Young RH, Scully RE: Stromal endometriosis of the uterine cervix: a variant of endometriosis that may simulate a sarcoma. Am J Surg Pathol 1990;14:449–455.
11 DeMay RM: The PapTest. Chicago, ASCP Press, 2005.
12 De Peralta-Venturino MN, Purslow MJ, Kini SR: Endometrial cells of the 'lower uterine segment' (LUS) in cervical smears obtained by endocervical brushings: a source of potential diagnostic pitfall. Diagn Cytopathol 1995;12:263–268; discussion 268–271.
13 Dhingra N, Punia RS, Radotra A, Mohan H: Arias-Stella reaction in upper genital tract in pregnant and non-pregnant women: a study of 120 randomly selected cases. Arch Gynecol Obstet 2007;276:47–52.
14 Ducatman BS, Wang HH, Jonasson JG, Hogan CL, Antonioli DA: Tubal metaplasia: a cytologic study with comparison to other neoplastic and non-neoplastic conditions of the endocervix. Diagn Cytopathol 1993;9:98–103; discussion 103–105.
15 Ersahin C, Huang M, Potkul RK, Hammadeh R, Salhadar A: Mesonephric adenocarcinoma of the vagina with a 3-year follow-up. Gynecol Oncol 2005;99:757–760.
16 Ganesan R, Ferryman SR, Waddell CA: Vaginal adenosis in a patient on Tamoxifen therapy: a case report. Cytopathol 1999;10:127–130.
17 Goodman A, Zukerberg LR, Nikrui N, Scully RE: Vaginal adenosis and clear cell carcinoma after 5-fluorouracil treatment for condylomas. Cancer 1991;68:1628–1632.
18 Hanau CA, Begley N, Bibbo M: Cervical endometriosis: a potential pitfall in the evaluation of glandular cells in cervical smears. Diagn Cytopathol 1997;16:274–280.

19 Hanselaar A, van Loosbroek M, Schuurbiers O, Helmerhosrt T, Bulten J, Bernheim J: Clear cell adenocarinoma of the vagina and cervix: an update of the Central Netherlands Registry showing twin age incidence peaks. Cancer 1997;79:2229–2236.
20 Hellen EA, Coghill SB, Clark JV: Prolapsed fallopian tube after abdominal hysterectomy: a report of the cytological findings. Cytopathology 1993;4: 181–185.
21 Hiroi H, Yasugi T, Matsumoto K, Fujii T, Watanabe T, Yoshikawa H, Taketani Y: Mucinous adenocarcinoma arising in a neovagina using the sigmoid colon thirty years after operation: a case report. J Surg Oncol 2001;77:61–64.
22 Hollowell ML, Goulart RA, Gang DL, Otis CN, Prior J, Sachs BF, Pantanowitz L: Cytologic features of müllerian papilloma of the cervix: mimic of malignancy. Diagn Cytopathol 2007;35:607–611.
23 Jiménez-Ayala M, Martínez Cabruja R, Esteban ML, Chinchilla C: Serous surface papillary carcinoma of the ovary metastatic to a cervical polyp: a case report. Acta Cytol 1996;40:765–769.
24 Lee KR: Atypical glandular cells in cervical smears from women who have undergone cone biopsy; a potential diagnostic pitfall. Acta Cytol 1993;37: 705–709.
25 Lu CH, Chang CC, Chang MC, Chen SJ, Jan YJ, Fu TF, Ho ES: Clinical parameters associated with unsatisfactory specimens of conventional cervical smears. Diagn Cytopathol 2010, Epub ahead of print.
26 Lui M, Boerner S: Arias-Stella reaction in a cervicovaginal smear of a woman undergoing infertility treatment: a case report. Diagn Cytopathol 2005; 32:94–96.
27 Lundeen SJ, Horwitz CA, Larson CJ, Stanley MW: Abnormal cervicovaginal smears due to endometriosis: a continuing problem. Diagn Cytopathol 2002;26:35–40.
28 Melnick S, Cole P, Anderson D, Herbst A: Rates and risks of diethylstilbestrol-related clear-cell adenocarcinoma of the vagina and cervix: an update. N Engl J Med 1987;316:514–516
29 Michael CW, Esfahani FM: Pregnancy-related changes: a retrospective review of 278 cervical smears. Diagn Cytopathol 1997;17:99–107.
30 Moore-Maxwell CA, Robboy SJ: Mucinous adenocarcinoma arising in rectovaginal fistulas associated with Crohn's disease. Gynecol Oncol 2004;93: 266–268.
31 Mudhar HS, Smith JH, Tidy J: Primary vaginal adenocarcinoma of intestinal type arising from an adenoma: case report and review of the literature. Int J Gynecol Pathol 2001;20:204–209.
32 Mulvany NJ, Surtees V: Cervical/vaginal endometriosis with atypia: a cytohistopathologic study. Diagn Cytopathol 1999;21:188–193.
33 Munkarah A, Malone JM Jr, Budev HD, Evans TN: Mucinous adenocarcinoma arising in a neovagina. Gynecol Oncol 1994;52:272–275.
34 Ngadiman S, Yang GH: Adenomyomatous lower uterine segment and endocervical polyps in cervicovaginal smears. Acta Cytol 1995;39:643–647.
35 Novotny DB, Maygarden SJ, Johnson DE, Frable WJ: Tubal metaplasia: a frequent potential pitfall in the cytologic diagnosis of endocervical glandular dysplasia on cervical smears. Acta Cytol 1992; 36:1–10.
36 Nucci MR, Young RH: Arias-Stella reaction of the endocervix: a report of 18 cases with emphasis on its varied histology and differential diagnosis. Am J Surg Pathol 2004;28:608–612.
37 Patten SF Jr: Diagnostic Cytopathology of the Uterine Cervix. Basel, Karger, 1978, pp 66–68.
38 Pisharodi LR, Jovanoska S: Spectrum of cytologic changes in pregnancy: a review of 100 abnormal cervicovaginal smears, with emphasis on diagnostic pitfalls. Acta Cytol 1995;39:905–908.
39 Ramdall RB, Wallach RC, Cangiarella J, Cai G, Elgert P, Simsir A, Levine P: Origin, frequency and clinical significance of glandular cells in liquid-based pap tests from patients posthysterectomy. Acta Cytol 2009;53:1–9.
40 Robboy SJ, Friedlander LM, Welch WR, Keh PC, Taft PD, Barnes AB, Scully RE, Herbst AL: Cytology of 575 young women with prenatal exposure to diethylstilbestrol. Obstet Gynecol 1976;48: 511–515.
41 Robboy SJ, Young RH, Welch WR, Truslow GY, Prat J, Herbst AL, Scully RE: Atypical vaginal adenosis and cervical ectropion: association with clear cell adenocarcinoma in diethylstilbestrol-exposed offspring. Cancer 1984;54:869–875.
42 Robboy SJ, Hill EC, Sandberg EC, Czernobilsky B: Vaginal adenosis in women born prior to the diethylstilbestrol era. Hum Pathol 1986;17:488–492.
43 Saitoh M, Hayasaka T, Ohmichi M, Kurachi H, Motoyama T: Primary mucinous adenocarcinoma of the vagina: possibility of differentiating from metastatic adenocarcinomas. Pathol Int 2005;55: 372–375.
44 Schlesinger C, Silverberg SG: Endocervical adenocarcinoma in situ of tubal type and its relation to atypical tubal metaplasia. Int J Gynecol Pathol 1999;18:1–4.
45 Schneider V: Arias-stella reaction of the endocervix: frequency and location. Acta Cytol 1981;25:224–228.
46 Sedlacek TV, Riva JM, Magen AB et al: Vaginal and vulvar adenosis: an unexpected side effect of CO_2 laser vaporisation. J Reprod Med 1990;35:995–1001.
47 Shah C, Pizer E, Veljovich DS, Drescher CW, Peters WA 3rd, Paley PJ: Clear cell adenocarcinoma of the vagina in a patient with vaginal endometriosis. Gynecol Oncol 2006;103:1130–1132.
48 Shidham VB, Rao RN, Machhi J, Chavan A: Microglandular hyperplasia has a cytomorphological spectrum overlapping with atypical squamous cells-cannot exclude high-grade squamous intraepithelial lesion (ASC-H). Diagn Cytopathol 2004; 30:57–61.
49 Staats PN, Clement PB, Young RH: Primary endometrioid adenocarcinoma of the vagina: a clinicopathologic study of 18 cases. Am J Surg Pathol 2007;31:1490–1501.
50 Szyfelbein WM, Baker PM, Bell DA: Superficial endometriosis of the cervix: a source of abnormal glandular cells on cervicovaginal smears. Diagn Cytopathol 2004;30:88–91.
51 Tambouret R, Pitman MB, Bell DA: Benign glandular cells in posthysterectomy vaginal smears. Acta Cytol 1998;42:1403–1408.
52 Valente PT, Schantz HD, Schultz M: Cytologic atypia associated with microglandular hyperplasia. Diagn Cytopathol 1994;10:326–331.
53 Veiga-Ferreira MM, Leiman G, Dunbar F, Margolius KA: Cervical endometriosis: facilitated diagnosis by fine needle aspiration cytologic testing. Am J Obstet Gynecol 1987;157:849–856.
54 Watanabe Y, Ueda H, Nozaki K, Kyoda A, Nakajima H, Hoshiai H, Noda K: Advanced primary clear cell carcinoma of the vagina not associated with diethylstilbestrol. Acta Cytol 2002;46:577–581.
55 Werner D, Wilkinson EJ, Ripley D, Yachnis A: Primary adenocarcinoma of the vagina with mucinous-enteric differentiation: a report of two cases with associated vaginal adenosis without history of diethylstilbestrol exposure. J Low Genit Tract Dis 2004;8:38–42.
56 World Health Organization Classification of Tumors: Tumors of the breast and female genital organs. Lyon, IARC Press, 2003.
57 Wolfendale M: Exfoliative cytology in a case of prolapsed fallopian tube. Acta Cytol 1980;24:545–548.
58 Yaghsezian H, Palazzo JP, Finkel GC, Carlson JA Jr, Talerman A: Primary vaginal adenocarcinoma of the intestinal type associated with adenosis. Gynecol Oncol 1992;45:62–65.
59 Young RH, Scully RE: Atypical forms of microglandular endocervical hyperplasia of the cervix simulating adenocarcinoma: a report of five cases and review of the literature. Am J Surg Pathol 1989;13:50–56.

Chapter 4

Cytopathology of Adenocarcinoma in situ of the Endocervix and Its Differential Diagnosis

4.1. Introduction

Although still rare if compared with the squamous lesions of the uterine cervix, pre-malignant and malignant lesions of the endocervical glandular epithelium seem to be increasing [19, 59]. This development may be partially the result of the decrease in the number of cases of invasive squamous cell carcinoma and cervical intraepithelial neoplasia (CIN), but there is also evidence for an absolute (not only relative) increase in some countries, particularly among young women [19]. As to the etiology, there is compelling evidence that – as in squamous lesions – that infection with HPV is a necessary initial event in the process of carcinogenesis. The occasional occurrence of carcinoma in situ of mixed, squamous and glandular types in close association supports this hypothesis. Interestingly, the spectrum of HPV-types seems to differ in that type 18 appears to be the most common virus found. As cofactors, hormonal influences have been postulated, in particular the long-term use of oral contraceptives. Whether this is of any significance is still debated.

There is agreement that adenocarcinoma in situ (AIS) is the precursor lesion of invasive adenocarcinoma of the endocervix [35, 42, 44, 64, 66]. On the other hand, there is controversy as to whether a recognizable precursor stage of AIS exists (endocervical dysplasia, low-grade cervical glandular intraepithelial neoplasia, endocervical glandular intraepithelial neoplasia (EGIN) grade 1 to 3, etc.). It seems that criteria for this postulated lesion are poorly defined and poorly reproducible, and it is unclear what biologic potential these lesions may have [64, 66]. Therefore, in daily practice most pathologists restrict their histologic diagnosis of preinvasive glandular lesions of the cervix to AIS [64]. In cytologic specimens, however, questionable cases of 'atypia' of endocervical type are categorized as 'atypical glandular cells'.

There is evidence that the glandular lesions of the endocervix are more difficult to detect in cytologic preparations [16, 19, 23, 24, 28, 33, 45, 50]. Part of the reason may be that these lesions are not as common as their squamous counterparts. But, there is also evidence that the criteria for AIS are less well established and less well known. It is therefore appropriate to outline in detail the morphologic appearance of AIS of the cervix in a chapter on its own.

4.2. Normal Endocervical Mucosa

The transition from the ectocervical squamous epithelium to the endocervical columnar epithelium is an important landmark because it defines the transformation zone which lies proximal to the original squamo-columnar junction. The endocervical canal is lined by a single layer of columnar cells of secretory type. In contrast to the protective function of the multilayered ectocervical squamous epithelium, the endocervical glandular epithelium provides a mucoid environment facilitating or preventing sperm penetration by variation of its composition depending upon the phase of the cycle. The presence of isolated ciliated cells in the cervix is normal and has been well documented by scanning electron microscopy. More recently, it has been shown that there are some differences in the cellular composition of the endocervical canal. The number of ciliated cells increases gradually towards the upper portions of the endocervical canal [5]. Similarly, the cells increasingly resemble endometrial cells. The lower uterine segment has been identified as source of diagnostic error. Particularly with cytologic sampling by brushing techniques, more cells of the higher portions of the endocervical canal are represented in the smear. The presence of crowded groups of ciliated cells (tubal metaplasia) or cells of the lower uterine segment may pose some problems in the differential diagnosis.

Glandular cells of secretory type in cytologic samples show the classic appearance of a honeycomb or strip pattern. The presence of endocervical glandular cells has been used as a quality marker for the adequacy of the cytologic sample [53]. However, evidence in longitudinal studies has shown that the detection rate of CIN is independent of the presence or absence of an endocervical component [32]. Therefore, the updated 2001 Bethesda System no longer classifies cervical smears according to the presence or absence of endocervical cells.

4.3. Benign and Reactive Changes

There are a number of lesions of the endocervical glandular epithelium which may cause considerable problems in differential diagnosis in a routine setting [37, 64]. Since the glandular epithelium is only 1 layer thick it is much more prone to reactive and inflammatory changes than the squamous epithelium. Most of these changes are non-specific. In rare instances specific inflammatory agents may be recognized in cervical smears (e.g. herpes, cytomegalovirus and follicular cervicitis). The now well established repair reaction of the uterine cervix is in most cases a reaction of the glandular and not the squamous epithelium [7]. It was described initially in 1971 by Bibbo, Keebler and Wied [7] and has stood the test of time [55, 63]. It is a useful diagnosis in cytologic practice although its histological counterpart is less well established, with the exception of the postoperative spindle cell nodule [26].

Metaplasia of squamous type is ubiquitous and essentially a daily diagnosis. Because of its squamous nature, it is not covered in this outline on glandular lesions. However, there are a number of other metaplastic reactions of glandular type which have been stressed in more recent times [11]. As already alluded to, ciliated cells are regularly observed in smears and sections of the cervix. As a reaction to irritation and inflammation, ciliated cells may proliferate focally leading to a lesion that has been termed tubal metaplasia [13, 22, 36, 37]. A more appropriate term would be 'ciliated cell metaplasia' since metaplasias are usually labeled according to cell type and not location. Tubal metaplasia usually occurs higher up in the endocervical canal [1] and has been recognized as an important differential diagnosis of repair and AIS [22, 36]. Other forms of metaplasia are 'transitional' [34, 61], 'oxyphylic' and 'endometrioid' [17, 21]. In particular, transitional cell metaplasia has been recently recognized as a lesion which may be confused with high-grade intraepithelial neoplasia. Murali et al. [34] described 6 cases of this entity, mainly in the postmenopausal age group, presenting with 3-dimensional clustering closely resembling high-grade squamous intraepithelial lesions. A focal 'streaming' pattern has been stressed as a criterion in the differential diagnosis.

Microglandular hyperplasia has been well known for some time and was initially related to usage of oral contraceptive pills. There have been a few reports on the cytologic appearance of microglandular hyperplasia [1, 56]. In my opinion, in daily practice this entity is exceedingly difficult to diagnose cytologically with certainty.

Table 4.1. Frequency of AIS in comparison with CIS: cervical conization 2000–2009

CIN 3, n	1,730
AIS, n	45
Ratio CIS:AIS	40:1

4.4. Adenocarcinoma in situ

Although initially already described in 1953 by Friedell and McKay [15], AIS came to prominence only in the last 30 years. There are now a number of excellent references on its clinical, colposcopic, histological and cytological presentation [2, 4, 8, 18, 27, 30, 33, 39, 41, 43, 45]. In particular, Australian and Japanese authors have shown considerable interest in this lesion.

AIS is a rare lesion. In my own material, in the 10-year period between 2000 and 2009, a total of 45 cases of AIS were diagnosed among 3,825 conization specimens. In the same period, 1,720 cases of CIN 3 were observed. That makes a CIN to AIS ratio of 40:1 (table 4.1). For practical considerations in daily routine work, it indicates that many cases of CIN are likely to be seen before a bona fide case of AIS is encountered. In a study from England in 2001 [14] the ratio of CIS to AIS was 50:1. The mean age in my material was 39 years, slightly higher than in the CIN 3 group, yet at least 12–15 years younger than patients with frank invasive carcinoma of the endocervix, giving support to the concept that AIS is the precursor of invasive disease. The simultaneous presence of AIS and CIS (so-called combined lesions)

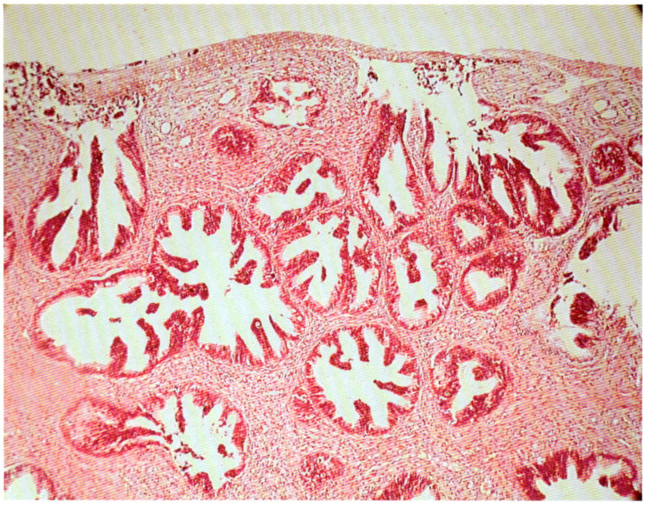

Fig. 4.1. Low-power view of AIS in a histologic section. Complex glandular pattern, no invasion, loss of surface epithelium.

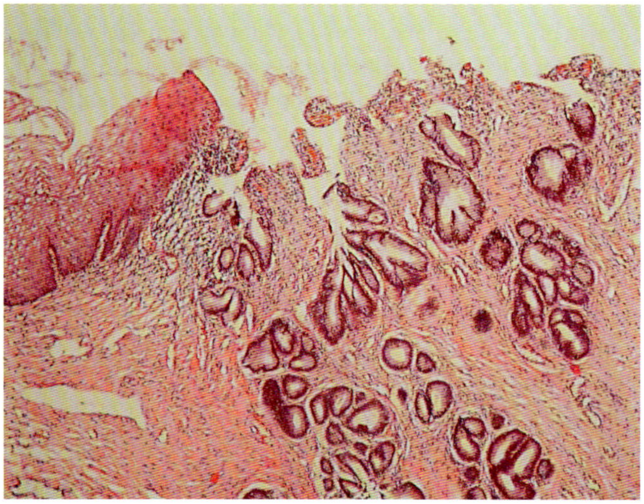

Fig. 4.2. Squamo-columnar junction with a focal AIS.

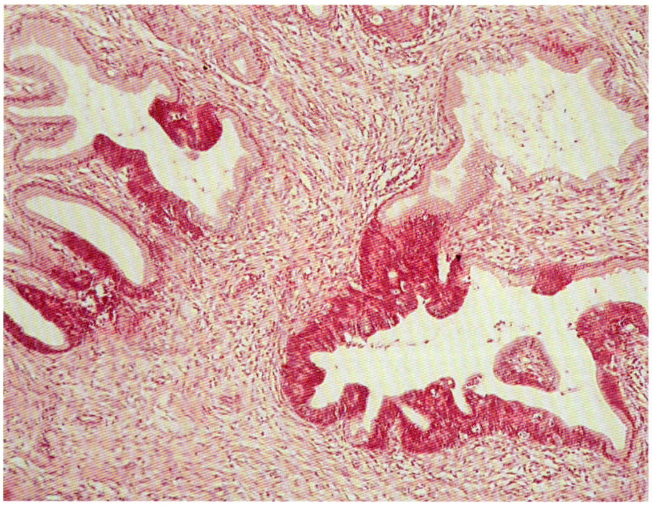

Fig. 4. 3. Focal AIS. Note the abrupt transition from normal glandular epithelium to the malignant epithelium.

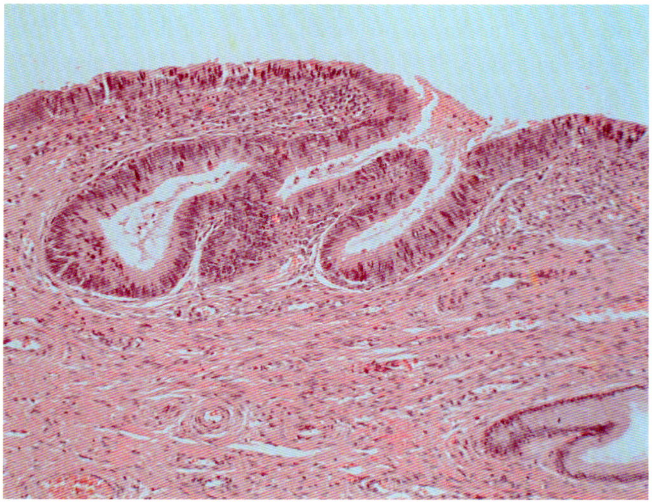

Fig. 4.4. Surface epithelium with pseudostratification, enlarged nuclei, loss of intracellular mucin and occasional mitoses.

was seen in 5 cases, making it only 10%. In other reports the presence of CIN components in AIS was seen in up to 50% [18, 57, 58, 65].

The histological appearance of AIS is fairly typical and straightforward if the diagnosis is considered. The endocervical glands are lined by enlarged cells with deep hyperchromasia of the nuclei and loss of mucin production in the cytoplasm. There is crowding of nuclei and pseudostratification, mitoses are common (fig. 4.1, 4.2). Frequently, the transition from the neighboring normal epithelium is abrupt, sometimes within a single gland (fig. 4.3). The chromatin is coarse, micronucleoli are evident (fig. 4.4). Apoptotic bodies may be seen often. Architecturally, there is cellular crowding within the glands with bridging and cribriform patterns (fig. 4.5, 4.6). To exclude microinvasion, a desmoplastic reaction in the stroma should be absent, although it may be difficult to ascertain because inflammatory reactions in the stroma of the endocervix are extremely common. A more significant criterion to exclude invasion is that the AIS occurs within the level of regular glands. If atypical glands are seen within

Table 4.2. Cytologic criteria for AIS

- Marked nuclear enlargement (factor 3 to 4)
- Three dimensional groupings ('hyperchromatic crowded groups')
- Marked hyperchromasia
- Coarse chromatin
- Mitoses and small nucleoli
- Architectural features:
  Epithelial gland in gland formation (rosettes)
  Stripped polar nuclei at the periphery (feathering)

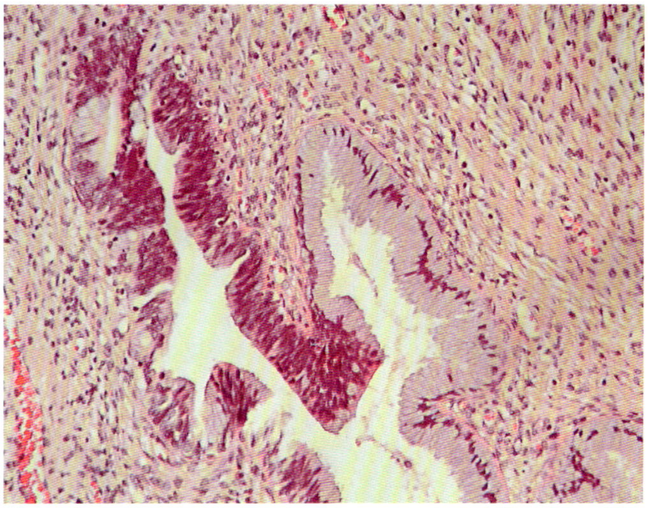

Fig. 4.5. Focal AIS within a gland. Note the difference in cell size, nuclear morphology and mucin formation between malignant and benign cells.

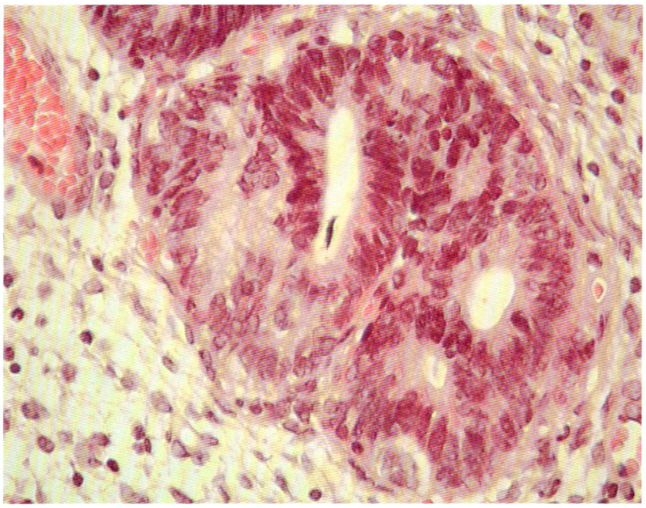

Fig. 4.6. High-power view of a complex gland in gland formation of AIS at higher power.

the cervical wall beyond the deepest situated gland, invasive disease has to be considered even if the atypicality is minor, as in the case of the so-called adenoma malignum [60]. In general, the exclusion of invasion is much more difficult in glandular than in squamous neoplasia.

Although most cases of AIS are of the usual endocervical type, some authors have claimed to recognize also endometrioid, serous and even tubal type [47] AIS in analogy to the World Health Organization subdivision of invasive adenocarcinoma. In the author's own experience, these lesions seem to be exceedingly rare and have no practical significance.

As already pointed out, I am in agreement with those authors who do not recognize a specific precursor lesion of AIS in clinical practice [64, 66]. Although changes of the glandular epithelium of a lesser degree than AIS are readily recognizable in histological and cytological material, such a diagnosis would only create insecurity and possibly overtreatment on the side of the clinician. I therefore do not use the diagnosis of low-grade intraepithelial neoplasia of glandular type in histological sections, and only rarely use a diagnosis of atypical glandular cells in cytological specimen.

Cytologically, a confident diagnosis of AIS requires a number of well established features [2, 8, 30, 41, 44]. Most importantly, the nuclei have to be markedly enlarged (by a factor of 3–4) compared with normal or reactive endocervical cells. Often, pale naked nuclei with considerable enlargement are observed in cytological smears. They cannot be taken as evidence of either endocervical origin or as a sign of AIS. It is prudent to scan the slide carefully to find better preserved areas and cells with remnants of cytoplasm to come to a definitive diagnosis. Often, these commonly occurring naked hypochromatic nuclei prove to be of squamous origin and are benign. Therefore, marked hyperchromasia and coarsening of the chromatin is essential for a diagnosis of AIS (table 4.2). Micronucleoli may be seen, as will be apoptotic bodies. Very important for the diagnosis are architectural features. Mostly, AIS presents as so-called hyperchromatic crowded groups with a 3-dimensional arrangement and prominent nuclear overlapping. Although feathering and rosette formation have been stressed as typical features, they are by no means found in all cases of AIS. Formation of rosettes are a cytological expression of the complex gland-in-gland structures seen in histology (fig. 4.7, 4.8). The feathering phenomenon shows peripheral palisading of oval nuclei, the rim of basal cytoplasm stripped

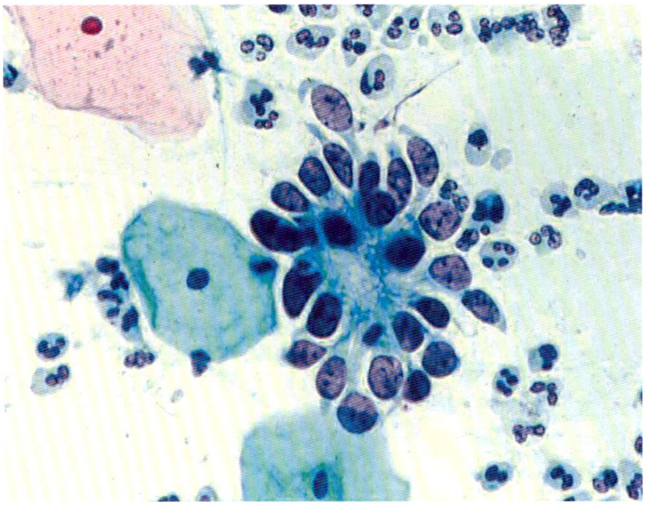

Fig. 4.7. Classic rosette formation of AIS. Note the marked enlargement of the nuclei with hyperchromasia.

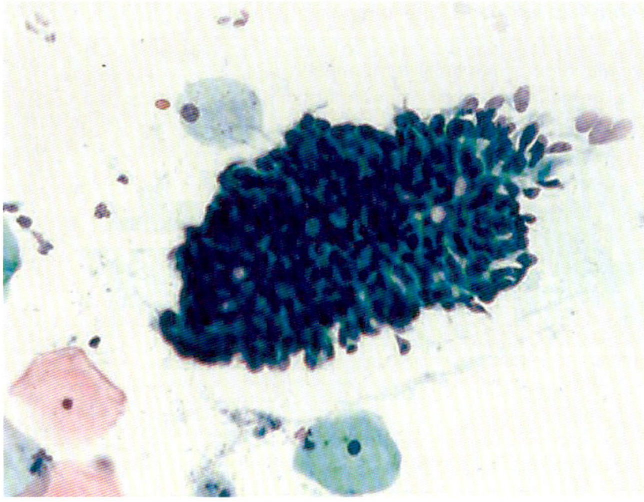

Fig. 4.9. Hyperchromatic crowded group of AIS. For a firm diagnosis, neighboring areas have to be evaluated.

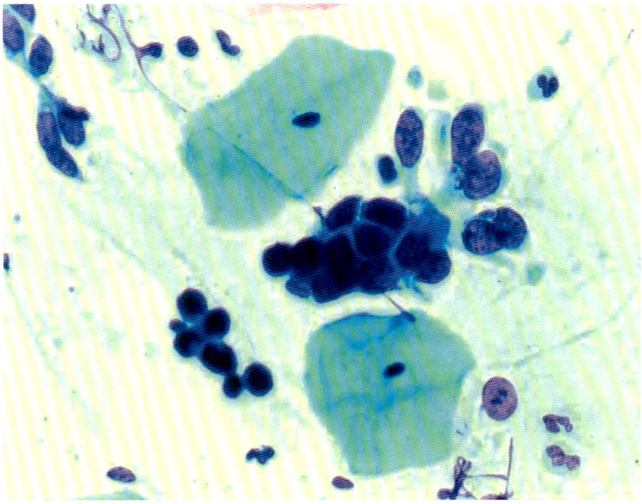

Fig. 4.8. Cells of AIS in small groups and as single cells.

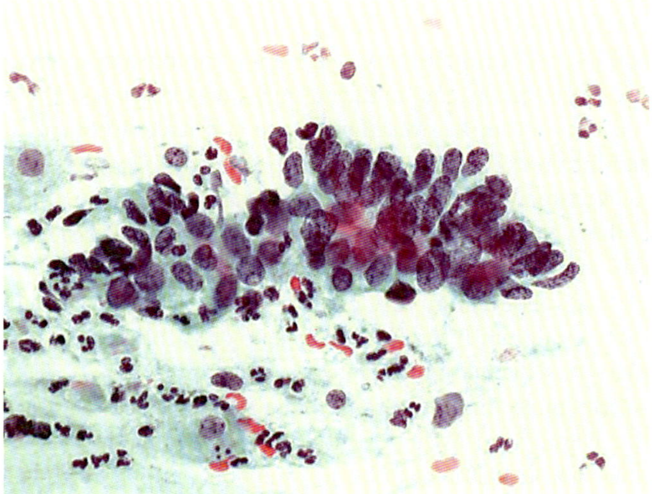

Fig. 4. 10. Cell cluster of AIS with peripheral palisading, there is marked hyperchromasia, nuclear enlargement and coarse chromatin.

off (fig. 4.9, 4.10). There have been single case reports of rare subtypes of AIS, but their frequency is so low and their criteria too indeterminate to draw general conclusions.

4.5. Clinical Management of AIS

If a firm diagnosis of AIS has been made cytologically, histological confirmation is mandatory. This may be either done by biopsy under colposcopic guidance or by conization. As already alluded to, in a substantial number of cases the final histological diagnosis will be CIN 3 [12, 52]. If AIS is confirmed histologically, further management does not differ from that of CIN. If invasion is excluded and the margins of resection are free, no further therapy is necessary [9, 39, 46, 51]. There has been considerable debate in the past [14] whether conization is sufficient in cases of AIS because suspected multifocality could involve the upper endocervical canal, requiring more aggressive therapy. With several large follow-up studies of conservative treatment of AIS [9, 51], there is now ample evidence that the recurrence rate is not higher than in CIN, confirming the morphologic observations that AIS develops – again as CIN – in the narrow area of the transformation zone at the squamo-columnar junction of the cervix.

4.6. Microinvasive Adenocarcinoma

More recently, the histologic criteria of a microinvasive version of adenocarcinoma have been established [18, 31, 38, 66]. Equally important, guidelines for the clinical management have been published based on several larger studies [20, 25, 54].

Histologically, there should be clear-cut evidence that malignant glands are seen outside the boundaries of the regular endocervical field [31, 66]. However, since the depth of distribution of regular endocervical glands is highly variable, the diagnosis may be difficult on occasion. Often, a desmoplastic reaction may be noticeable. Necrosis is absent. Östör et al. [38] summarized the histological criteria in a landmark study of 77 cases in 1997. Cytologically, microinvasion of cervical adenocarcinoma cannot be made with any degree of certainty, although several publications dealt with the topic as early as 1975 [3, 18, 27, 40]. The cells are enlarged, have hyperchromatic nuclei and prominent nucleoli. They occur in 3-dimensional clusters and may be accompanied by focal areas of necrosis.

Management of microinvasive adenocarcinoma has been controversial for some time. Because of fear of multifocality within the endocervical canal, initial recommendations were hysterectomy. Within recent years several larger studies have appeared documenting that the treatment could be the same as in microinvasive squamous carcinoma of the cervix [25]. If preservation of fertility is desired, the margins of resection are free and there are no risk factors such as lymphoid or vascular invasion, conization could be sufficient treatment. Close follow-up should be mandatory.

4.7. CIN 3 Mimics AIS

It is a well-known fact that in approximately half of cases with a cytological diagnosis of AIS, the ultimate histological diagnosis will be a high-grade squamous lesion [12]. In particular, CIN 3 with extensive involvement of endocervical glands will present, with numerous hyperchromatic crowded groups mimicking a glandular appearance [52]. Therefore, a 3-dimensional appearance of cellular groupings should not lead automatically to a suspicion of glandular origin. The more vigorous sampling techniques of brush and spatula tend to remove larger tissue fragments in 3-dimensional clusters. It appears that with involvement of endocervical glands by CIN 3, atypical squamous cells are removed in particularly large groupings. In the cytological smear these clusters appear glandlike, but a closer scrutiny of single cells in the neighborhood will demonstrate typical squamous features such as central position of the nucleus, sharp cell borders and transparent cytoplasm. It should be noted, however, that the combined occurrence of CIS and AIS may occasionally confuse the picture [9].

4.8. Pregnancy Changes

The hormonal changes of pregnancy usually lead to an eversion of the glandular epithelium onto the ectocervix and to edema and softening of the cervix. Therefore, bioptic procedures and even taking smears usually result in easy bleeding during pregnancy. There are a few changes specific for pregnancy which may cause differential diagnostic problems. Decidualization of the cervical stroma is common during later pregnancy and my lead to exfolation of decidual cells [49]. They are enlarged and possess prominent nuclei with nucleoli. Similarly, endocervical glandular cells may alter their appearance during pregnancy. The Arias-Stella reaction is a regular observation in endometrial glands and may also be occasionally present in the endocervix [48]. Cells are massively enlarged and may mimic malignancy. Thus, the diagnosis of adenocarcinoma during pregnancy should therefore be made with great caution.

4.9. The Vaginal Cuff

Even after hysterectomy, glandular cells may occasionally be observed in vaginal smears [6]. This paradoxical situation has been reported and discussed lately in the literature. It was therefore included in the new Bethesda terminology of 2001. Sources for glandular cells may be adenosis, which is exceedingly rare in non-diethylstilbestrol-exposed females, tubal prolapse, endometriosis, recto-vaginal fistula or goblet cell metaplasia. Personally, I have observed several cases of prolapsed fallopian tube which caused considerable differential diagnostic problems [62]. Finally, metastases of adenocarcinomas of pelvic or extrapelvic origin may exfoliate after hysterectomy [29], most common is an involvement of the vaginal cuff by endometrial adenocarcinoma.

References

1 Alvarez-Santin C, Sica A, Rodriguez M, Feijo A, Garrido G: Microglandular hyperplasia in the uterine cervix: cytologic diagnosis in cervical smears. Acta Cytol 1999;43:110–113.

2 Ayer B, Pacey F, Greenberg M, Bousfield L: The cytologic diagnosis of adenocarcinoma in situ of the cervix uteri and related lesions. I. Adenocarcinoma in situ. Acta Cytol 1987;31:397–411.

3 Ayer B, Pacey F, Greenberg M: The cytologic diagnosis of adenocarcinoma in situ of the cervix uteri and related lesions. II. Microinvasive adenocarcinoma. Acta Cytol 1988;32:318–324.

4 Betsill WL, Clark AH: Early endocervical glandular neoplasia: I. Histomorphology and cytomorphology. Acta Cytol 1986;30:115–126.

5 Babkowski RC, Wilbur DC, Rutkowski MA, Facik MS, Bonfiglio TA: The effects of endocervical canal topography, tubal metaplasia and high canal sampling on the cytologic presentation of non-neoplastic endocervical cells. Am J Clin Pathol 1996;105:403–410.

6 Bewtra C: Columnar cells in post-hysterectomy vaginal smears. Diagn Cytopathol 1992;8:342–345.

7 Bibbo M, Keebler CM, Wied GL: The cytologic diagnosis of tissue repair in the female genital tract. Acta Cytol 1971;15:133–137.

8 Biscotti CV, Gero MA, Toddy SM, Fischler DF, Easley KA: Endocervical adenocarcinoma in situ: an analysis of cellular features. Diagn Cytopathol 1997;17:326–332.

9 Bull-Phelps SL, Garner El, Walsh CS, Gehrig PA, Miller DS, Schorge JO: Fertility sparing surgery in 101 women with adenocarcinoma in situ of the cervix. Gynecol Oncol 2007;107:316–319.

10 Clark AH, Betsill WL: Early endocervical glandular neoplasia. II. Morphometric analysis of the cells. Acta Cytol 1986;30:127–134.

11 Dlott JS, Dlott TR, Matthews TH, O'Connor DM: Endocervical metaplasias and their asociation with glandular and squamous abnormalities. J Lower Genit Tract Dis 1999;3:77–82.

12 Drijkoningen M, Meertens B, Lauweryns J: High grade squamous intraepithelial lesion (CIN 3) with extension into the endocervical clefts: difficulty of cytologic differentiation from adenocarcinoma in situ. Acta Cytol 1996;40:889–894.

13 Ducatman B, Wang HH, Jonasson JG, Hogan CL, Antonioli DA: Tubal metaplasia: a cytologic study with comparison to other neoplastic and non-neoplastic conditions of the endocervix. Diagn Cytopathol 1993;9:98–105.

14 Etherington IJ, Luesley DM: Adenocarcinoma in situ of the cervix: controversies in diagnosis and treatment. J Low Genit Tract Dis 2001;5:94–98.

15 Friedell GH, McKay DG: Adenocarcinoma in situ of the endocervix. Cancer 1953;6:887–897.

16 Geldenhuys I, Murray ML: Sensitivity and specificity of the Pap smear for glandular lesions of the cervix and endometrium. Acta Cytol 2007;51:47–50.

17 Hanau CA, Begley N, Bibbo M: Cervical endometriosis: a potential pitfall in the evaluation of glandular cells in cervical smears. Diagn Cytopathol 1997;16:274–280.

18 Hayes MMM, Matisic JP, Chen CJ, Mohamed A, Anderson GH, LeRiche JC, Amy R: Cytological aspects of uterine cervical adenocarcinoma, adenosquamous carcinoma and combined adenocarcinoma-squamous carcinoma: appraisal of diagnostic criteria for in situ versus invasive lesions. Cytopathology 1997;8:397–408.

19 Herbert A, Singh N, Smith H: Adenocarcinoma of the uterine cervix compared with squamous cell carcinoma: a 12-year study in Southampton and South-West Hampshire. Cytopathology 2001;12:26–36.

20 Hirai, Y, Takeshima N, Tate S, Akiyama F, Furuta R, Hasumi K: Early invasive cervical adenocarcinoma: its potential for nodal metastasis or recurrence. BJOG 2003;110:241–246.

21 Hirschowitz L, Eckford SD, Phillpotts B, Midwinter A: Cytological changes associated with tubo-endometrioid metaplasia of the cervix. Cytopathology 1994;5:1–8.

22 Jonasson JG, Wang HH, Antonioli DA, Ducatman BS: Tubal metaplasia of the uterine cervix: a prevalence study in patients with gynecologic pathologic findings. Int J Gynecol Pathol 1992;11:89–95.

23 Kalir T, Simsir A, Demopoulos HB, Demopoulos RI: Obstacles to the early detection of endocervical adenocarcinoma. Int J Gynecol Pathol 2005;24:399–403.

24 Kane JF, Granter SR, Trask CE, Hogan CL, Lee KR: Papanicolaou smear sensitivity for the detection of adenocarcinoma of the cervix. Cancer (Cancer Cytopathol) 2001;93:8–15.

25 Kasamatsu T, Okada S, Tsuda H, Shiromizu K, Yamada T, Tsunematsu R, Ohmi K: Early invasive adenocarcinoma of the uterine cervix: criteria for non-radical surgical treatment. Gynecol Oncol 2002;85:327–332.

26 Kay S, Schneider V: Reactive spindle cell nodule of the endocervix simulating uterine sarcoma. Int J Gynecol Pathol 1985;4:255–257.

27 Keyhani-Rofagha S, Brewer S, Prokorym P: Comparative cytologic findings of in situ and invasive adenocarcinoma of the uterine cervix. Diagn Cytopathol 1995;12:120–125.

28 Kinney W, Sawaya GF, Sung HY, Kearney KA, Miller M, Hiatt RA: Stage at diagnosis and mortality in patients with adenocarcinoma and adenosquamous carcinoma of the uterine cervix diagnosed as a consequence of cytologic screening. Acta Cytol 2003;47:167–171.

29 Kumar A, Schneider V: Metastases to the uterus from extrapelvic primary tumors. Int J Gynecol Pathol 1983;2:134–140.

30 Laverty CR, Farnsworth A, Thurlow J, Bowditch R: The reliability of a cytological prediction of cervical adenocarcinoma in situ. Aust NZ J Obstet Gynaecol 1988;28:307–312.

31 Lee KR, Flynn CE: Early invasive adenocarcinoma of the cervix. Cancer 2000;89:1048–1055.

32 Mitchell HS: Longitudinal analysis of histologic high-grade disease after negative cervical cytology according to endocervical status. Cancer Cytopathol 2001;93:237–240.

33 Mitchell H, Hocking J, Saville M: Cervical cytology screening history of women diagnosed with adenocarcinoma in situ of the cervix: a case control study. Acta Cytol 2004;48:595–600.

34 Murali R, Loughman NT, Pagliuso J, McKenzie PR, Watson GF, Earls P, Russell P: Cytological features of transitional cell metaplasia of the lower female genital tract. Pathology 2010;42:113–118.

35 Negri G, Egarter-Vigl E, Kasal A, et al: p16 ink4a is a useful marker for the diagnosis of adenocarcinoma of the cervix uteri and its precursors: an immunohistochemical study with immunocytochemical correlations. Am J Surg Pathol 2003;27:187–193.

36 Novotny D, Maygarden S, Johnson DE, Frable WJ: Tubal metaplasia: a frequent potential pitfall in the cytologic diagnosis of endocervical glandular dysplasia on cervical smears. Acta Cytol 1992;36:1–10.

37 Nucci MR: Symposium part III: tumor-like glandular lesions of the uterine cervix. Int J Gynecol Pathol 2002;21:347–359.

38 Östör AG, Rome R, Quinn M: Microinvasive adenocarcinoma of the cervix: a clinicopathologic study of 77 women. Obstet Gynecol 1997;89: 88–93.

39 Östör AG; Duncan A, Quinn M, Rome R: Adenocarcinoma in situ of the uterine cervix: an experience with 100 cases. Gynecol Oncol 2000;79:207–210.

40 Quizilbash AH: In situ and microinvasive adenocarcinoma of the uterine cervix: a clinical, cytologic and histologic study of 14 cases. Am J Clin Pathol 1975;64:155–170.

41 Renshaw AA, Mody DR, Lozano RL, et al: Detection of adenocarcinoma in situ of the cervix in Papanicoloaou tests. Arch Pathol Lab Med 2004;128:153–157.

42 Riethdorf L, Riethdorf S, Lee KR, et al: Human papillomaviruses, expression of p16 and early endocervical glandular neoplasia. Hum Pathol 2002;33:899–904.

43 Pacey NF, Ayer B, Greenberg M: The cytologic diagnosis of adenocarcinoma in situ of the cervix uteri and related lesions. III. Pitfalls in diagnosis. Acta Cytol 1988;32:325–330.

44 Pacey NF: Glandular neoplasms of the uterine cervix; in M Bibbo (ed): Comprehensive Cytopathology. Philadelphia, Saunders, 1991, pp 231–256.

45 Ruba S, Schooland M, Allpress S, et al: Adenocarcinoma in situ of the uterine cervix: screening and diagnostic errors in Papanicolaou smears. Cancer (Cancer Cytopathol) 2004;102:280–287.

46 Salani R, Puri I, Bristow RE: Adenocarcinoma in situ of the uterine cervix: a metaanalysis of 1,278 patients evaluating the predictive value of conization margin status. Am J Obstet Gynecol 2009;200:182, e1–e5.

47 Schlesinger C, Silverberg SG: Endocervical adenocarcinoma in situ of tubal type and its relation to atypical tubal metaplasia. Int J Gynecol Pathol 1999;18:1–4.
48 Schneider V: Arias-Stella reaction of the endocervix: frequency and location. Acta Cytol 1981; 25:224–228.
49 Schneider V, Barnes LA: Ectopic decidual reaction of the uterine cervix: frequency and cytologic presentation. Acta Cytol 1981;25:616–622.
50 Schooland M, Segal A, Allpress S, et al: Adenocarcinoma in situ of the cervix. sensitivity of detection by cervical smear. Cancer (Cancer Cytopathol) 2004;102:280–287.
51 Schorge JO, Lea JS, Ashfaq R: Post-conization surveillance of cervical adenocarcinoma in situ: a prospective trial. J Reprod Med 2003:48:751–755.
52 Selvaggi SM: Cytologic features of squamous cell carcinoma in situ involving endocervical glands in endocervical cytobrush specimens. Acta Cytol 1994;38:687–692.
53 Sidawy MK, Tabbara SO, Silverberg SG: Should we report cervical smears lacking endocervical componenet as inadequate? Diagn Cytopathol 1992;8: 567–570.
54 Teshima S, Shimosata Y, Kishi K, Kasumatsu T, Ohmi K, Uei Y: Early stage adenocarcinoma of the uterine cervix: histopathologic analysis with consideration of histogenesis. Cancer 1985;56:167–172.
55 Ueki M, Ueda M, Kurokawa A: Cytologic study of the tissue repair cells of the uterine cervix with special reference to their origin. Acta Cytol 1992; 36:310–318.
56 Valente PT, Schantz HD, Schultz M: Cytologic atypia associated with microglandular hyperplasia of the cervix. Diagn Cytopathol 1994;10:326–331.
57 van Aspert-van Erp AJM, van't Hof-Grootenboer AB, Brugal G, Voojis PG: Endocervical columnar cell intraepithelial neoplasia. I. Discriminating cytomorphologic criteria. Acta Cytol 1995;39:1199–1215.
58 van Aspert-van Erp AJM, van't Hof-Grootenboer AB, Brugal G, Voojis PG: Endocervical columnar cell intraepithelial neoplasia. II. Grades of expression of cytomorphologic criteria. Acta Cytol 1995; 39:1199–1215, 1216–1232.
59 Vesterinen E, Forrs M, Nieminen U: Increase of cervical adenocarcinoma: a report of 520 cases of cervical carcinoma including 112 tumors with glandular elements. Gynecol Oncol 1989;33:49–53.
60 Vogelsang PJ, Nguyen GK, Honore LH: Exfoliative cytology of adenoma malignum (minimal deviation adenocarcinoma) of the uterine cervix. Diagn Cytopathol 1995;13:146–150.
61 Weir MM, Bell D, Young RH: Transitional cell metaplasia of the uterine cervix and vagina: an underrecognized lesion that may be confused with high grade dysplasia. A report of 59 cases. Am J Surg Pathol 1997;21:510–517.
62 Wheelock JB, Schneider V, Goplerud D: Prolapsed Fallopian tube masquerading as adenocarcinoma of the vagina in a postmenopausal woman. Gynecol Oncol 1985;21:369–375.
63 Yelverton CL, Bentley RC, Olenick S, et al: Epithelial repair of the uterine cervix: assessment of morphologic features and correlations with cytologic diagnosis. Int J Gynecol Pathol 1996; 15:338–344.
64 Young RH: Simple clefts, complex problems: reflections on glandular lesions of the uterine cervix. Int J Gynecol Pathol 2002;21:212–216.
65 Zafar N, Balazs L, Benstein BD: Synchronous high-grade squamous intraepithelial lesion and adenocarcinoma in situ of cervix in a young woman presenting with hyperchromatic crowded groups in the cervical cytology specimen: report of a case. Diagn Cytopathol 2008:36:823–826.
66 Zaino R: Symposium part I: adenoca in situ, glandular dysplasia, and early invasive adenocarcinoma of the uterine cervix. Int J Gynecol Pathol 2002;21:314–326.

Chapter 5

Cytopathology of the Malignant Invasive Lesions of the Endocervix

5.1. Introduction

There is general evidence that the incidence of the adenocarcinoma of the endocervix (EA) has been rising, particularly in the lower age groups. The increase is multinational, covering the USA, northern Europe and other Western countries. There has been both an absolute and relative increase of EA compared with squamous cell carcinoma (SCC), over the past 2 decades: EA makes up between 15 and 25% of invasive carcinoma [19]. The trends are generally restricted to younger women under 25.

Almost 60% of EA are associated with squamous intraepithelial lesions (SIL) or invasive squamous carcinoma. EA usually develops slowly, but unfortunately with late clinical symptoms. Between 10 and 20% of cases are asymptomatic when the invasive state has been diagnosed and late detection is often observed. The most frequent symptom is abnormal vaginal bleeding.

Available data show that EA is related to the number of partners and to lower age at first intercourse, suggesting a role for sexually transmitted viral factors. It is widely accepted that human papillomavirus (HPV) can be found in most cases of EA, as well as of endocervical adenocarcinoma in situ (AIS), and also that types 18 and 16 are found in most cases, with a frequency of 80%. In contrast with SCC, HPV_{18} is more common than HPV_{16}.

A second risk factor seems to be oral contraceptives, although a few studies have suggested that the risk is only increasing for certain types of adenocarcinoma, such as villoglandular adenocarcinoma and adenosquamous carcinoma [11]. A case control review by the Silverberg Group [15] shows that the use of contraceptives seems to be positively and significantly associated with EA. It is accepted that a consistent association exists between current oral contraceptive use and AIS.

Finally, some authors have suggested similarities with the epidemiology of endometrial adenocarcinoma. An association with obesity seems clear, while it is more difficult to interpret a possible relationship with hypertension and diabetes. If this suggestion is proven, EA would appear to share characteristics with both adenosquamous carcinoma and endometrial adenocarcinoma.

5.2. Types of Malignant Invasive Lesions of the Endocervix

For didactic purposes we have classified these malignant lesions as follows:

- Invasive endocervical adenocarcinoma. The WHO classification of the glandular tumors is presented in table 5.1.
- Uncommon carcinomas of the cervix.
- Metastatic tumors to the cervix.

5.3. Invasive Endocervical Adenocarcinoma

5.3.1. Early Invasive Adenocarcinoma

Early invasive adenocarcinoma (EIA) refers to a glandular neoplasm in which the extent of stromal invasion is so minimal that the risk of local lymph node metastasis is negligible. It is also called microinvasive adenocarcinoma. This concept is controversial. The current 1995 FIGO staging omits specific reference to glandular lesion in stage IA

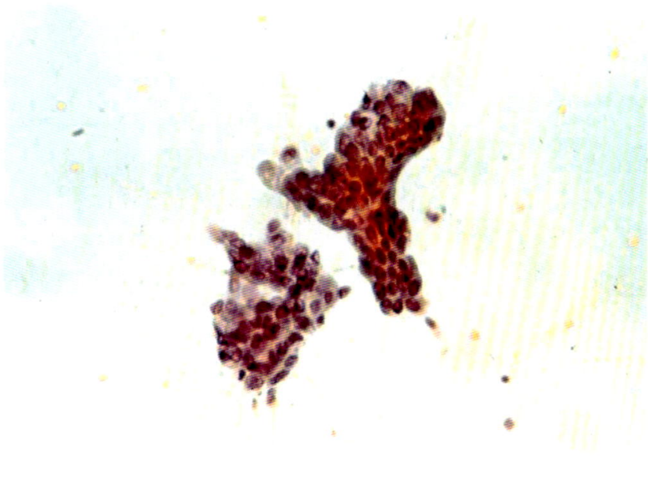

Fig. 5.9. Minimal deviation variant of endocervical adenocarcinoma shows cells with slight atypia, difficult to differentiate from benign endocervical cells.

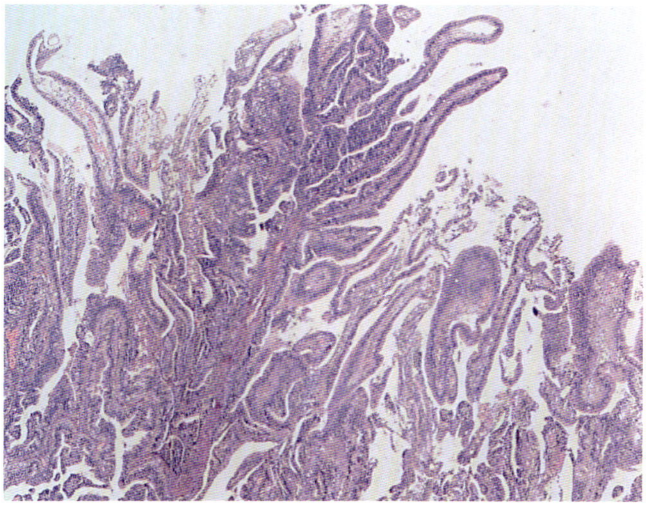

Fig. 5.10. Villoglandular adenocarcinoma presents a complex branching papillary process with mildly atypical columnar cells.

Some clues to achieve the diagnosis are the presence of a large indurate mass on clinical or colposcopic examination, glands penetrating deeply into the cervical wall and a marked variability in gland size and shape in the histological examination [15].

5.3.3. Villoglandular Adenocarcinoma

Concept. Villoglandular adenocarcinoma (VGA) is a well differentiated adenocarcinoma with a frond-like pattern resembling villoglandular adenoma of the colon. This tumor may not be invasive and when it is, it has pushing borders [17]. The term VGA should be reserved for this pure form, but not if only part of the tumor shows villoglandular growth [18]. In a small biopsy we should only suggest a possible VGA. For a definitive diagnosis we need a conization or a hysterectomy specimen. VGA occurs predominantly in young women and has an excellent prognosis. An association with oral contraceptives and high risk HPV types (mostly HPV_{16} and HPV_{18}) has been suggested [9].

Histological Features. It presents a complex branching papillary process with papillae and glands lined by stratified, mildly atypical columnar cells, some of which contain mucin. The adjacent epithelium often shows AIS (fig. 5.10).

Cytological Features. The cytological features are as follows:

- Arrangement. Large slender papillary and cohesive branching epithelial sheets with smooth borders and a lack of feathering edges. Single, intact atypical cells are sparse, but naked nuclei may be numerous [5] (fig. 5.11).
- Neoplastic cells. Atypia is mild to moderate. The nuclei are uniform with inconspicuous or absent nucleoli. Mitoses are infrequent.

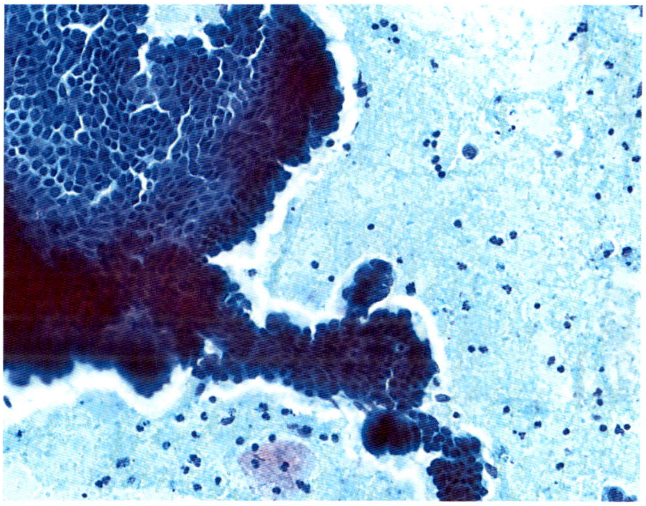

Fig. 5.11. Villoglandular adenocarcinoma is frequently not diagnosed cytologically, but suggestive features are a papillary architecture and little cytologic atypia.

The VGA is frequently not diagnosed cytologically, but suggestive features are villous fronds, true papillae with fibrovascular cores and little cytological atypia. A helpful clinical sign is the description of an exofytic tumor.

Differential Diagnosis. A major problem in the cytological diagnosis of VGA is misinterpretation of the tumor cells

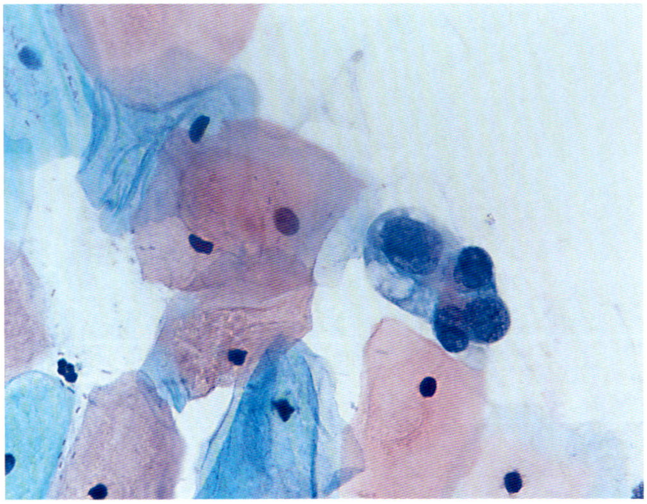

Fig. 5.12. Endometrioid adenocarcinoma of the cervix must be distinguished from the more common adenocarcinoma of the endometrium.

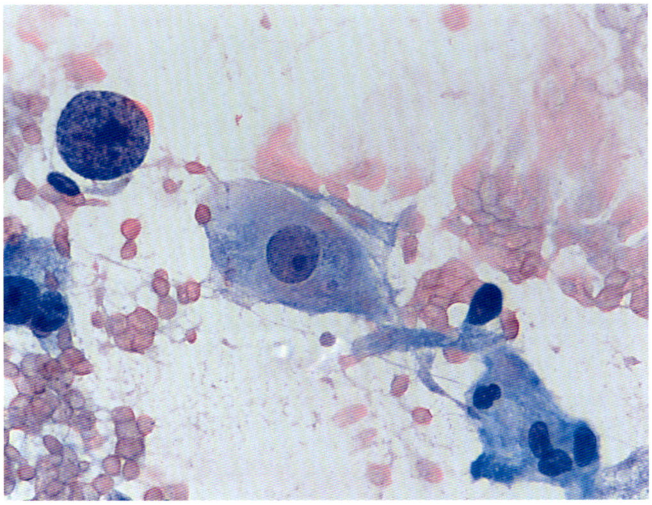

Fig. 5.13. Clear cell adenocarcinoma shows a large, atypical nucleus and abundant vacuolated or clear cytoplasm. Naked nuclei are usually present.

as benign, derived for example from endocervical polyps. Reactive endocervical changes usually present some degree of atypia with prominent nucleoli and absence of papillary configuration. Endometrial cells may be sampled by brushing, but benign tubular glands with stromal fragments and vessels are characteristic. VGA may be confused with in situ tumors such as squamous carcinoma in situ involving endocervical glands or AIS. Palisading nuclear arrangement with feathering edges of epithelial cells are typically seen in AIS. Other subtypes of EA should pose fewer difficulties. Clear cell, serous and the common endocervical adenocarcinoma present a greater degree of nuclear atypia. Endometrial adenocarcinomas are HPV negative [15].

5.3.4. Endometrioid Adenocarcinoma of the Cervix

This is morphologically identical to the endometrial counterpart. It usually arises at the squamous-columnar junction from reserve cells, but rarely arises in cervical endometriosis.

Histology. It presents the same features as an endometrioid adenocarcinoma of the endometrium, although squamous elements are less common. The tumors are usually well differentiated with no intracellular mucin and tall columnar cells, arranged perpendicular to the base of the glands [15].

Cytology. The tumor sheds loose clusters of small cells with eccentric nuclei, micronucleoli, and scant cytoplasm. Peripheral palisading or feathering of the nuclei are not seen (fig. 5.12).

Differential Diagnosis. The major problem is the differentiation from an endometrioid adenocarcinoma extending into the cervix from the endometrium. It may require a hysterectomy specimen for final diagnosis. Immunohistochemistry may be an important tool [15].

5.3.5. Clear-Cell Adenocarcinoma

Clear-cell adenocarcinoma (CCA) of the endocervix has histological and cytological features identical to the more common CCA of the ovary, endometrium and vagina.

Although it can occur sporadically, it was more common in daughters of women who took diethylstilbestrol (DES) during pregnancy, with a peak incidence between 14 to 22 years. There is a second peak at 70 years. The frequency of this tumor has decreased following the withdrawal of DES from the market in the last 40 years.

Histology. CCA presents tubulocystic, solid, and papillary patterns, with clear and hobnail cells and atypical nuclei with prominent nucleoli.

Cytology. The arrangement of the neoplastic cells may be in sheets, clusters, papillae or as single cells. They have large, pleomorphic nuclei with prominent nucleoli and abundant finely vacuolated or clear cytoplasm. Naked nuclei may be numerous (fig. 5.13).

Diagnosis. FIGO tumor stage I was preceded more frequently by cytology than the higher tumor stages. Consequently the majority of CCA cases can be detected at an early stage by yearly clinical and cytological examination, which must comprise cervical as well as vaginal sampling. Since CCA may also occur in postmenopausal women, regular cytologic examination of DES-exposed women must be continued after menopause.

Differential Diagnosis. The diagnosis of primary CCA should be made only when spread from the ovary, endometrium and vagina has been excluded. SCCs may present clear cells but usually show focal keratinization. Arias-Stella reaction shows atypical cells with abundant clear cytoplasm. A clinical history of pregnancy is essential to avoid a false-positive diagnosis.

5.3.6. Serous Adenocarcinoma

Serous adenocarcinoma (SA) of the endocervix has histological and cytological features identical to SA of the ovary and endometrium, where they are more common. Its behavior is aggressive, with lymph node involvement and extragenital spread [22].

Histology. SA shows a complex pattern of papillae with cellular budding and the frequent presence of psammoma bodies.

Cytological Patterns. SA is a high-grade tumor with large, pleomorphic cells with macronucleoli. Papillary structures are common. Psammoma bodies are generally not seen in cytologic specimens (fig. 5.14).

Differential Diagnosis. The diagnosis of primary SA should be made only when spread from the ovary, fallopian tube, endometrium and peritoneum has been excluded. Villoglandular adenocarcinoma also has papillae, but the cells are well-differentiated. Some papillae may also be seen in CCA; both CCA and SA are high-grade tumors, although a large, clear cytoplasm is only seen in the former [21].

5.4. Uncommon Carcinomas of the Cervix

The WHO classification includes as uncommon carcinomas of the cervix, epithelial tumors other than those of squamous or glandular types: adenosquamous carcinoma, glassy-cell carcinoma variant, adenoid cystic carcinoma, adenoid basal carcinoma and neuroendocrine tumors.

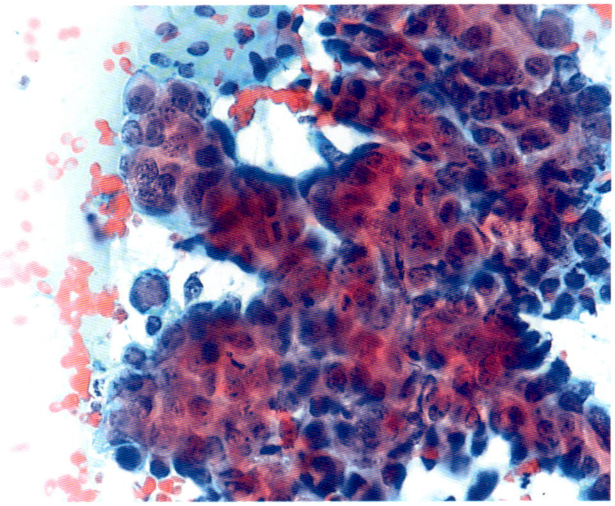

Fig. 5.14. Serous adenocarcinoma shows a papillary architecture with high-grade tumor cells.

5.4.1. Adenosquamous Carcinoma of the Cervix

Adenosquamous carcinoma of the cervix (ADSC) is defined as a tumor in which both squamous and glandular malignant features are evident without special stains [15]. It has an unfavorable prognosis and is usually HPV DNA+.

Cytology. ADSC shows mixed glandular and squamous malignant cells, and tumor diathesis. The glandular component is usually of the endocervical type. Malignant squamous elements can be keratinized or non-keratinized SCC (fig. 5.15). Both components are difficult to distinguish in a poorly differentiated pattern.

5.4.2. Glassy Cell Carcinoma Variant

Glassy cell carcinoma (GCC) is a poorly differentiated variant of ADSC, described by Glucksmann and Cherry in 1956 [6]. The tumor occurs in young women, grows rapidly, develops frequent distant metastasis and responds poorly to radiotherapy. The absence of estrogen and progesterone receptors suggests that this tumor would not be hormonal dependant and that these patients can be safely treated with hormonal replacement therapy [1].

Histology. GCC presents sheets and nests of malignant cells with scanty intervening stroma and a prominent eosinophilic and plasma cell infiltrate. The cells are large, with distinct cell borders and a ground-glass cytoplasm. Nuclei are large and have macronucleoli. Rare fields of squamous or

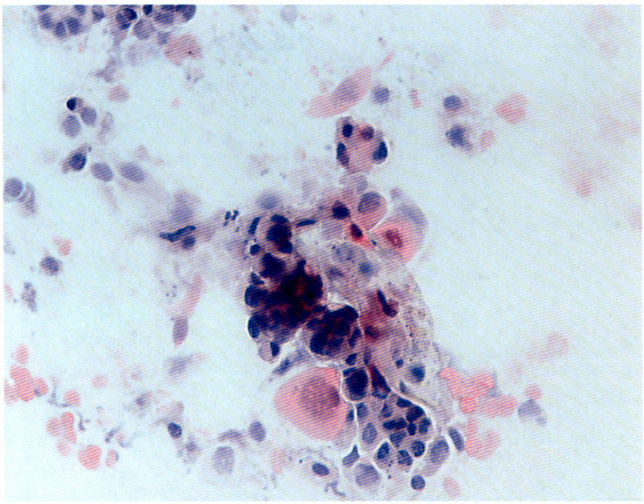

Fig. 5.15. Adenosquamous carcinoma of the cervix shows mixed glandular and squamous malignant cells.

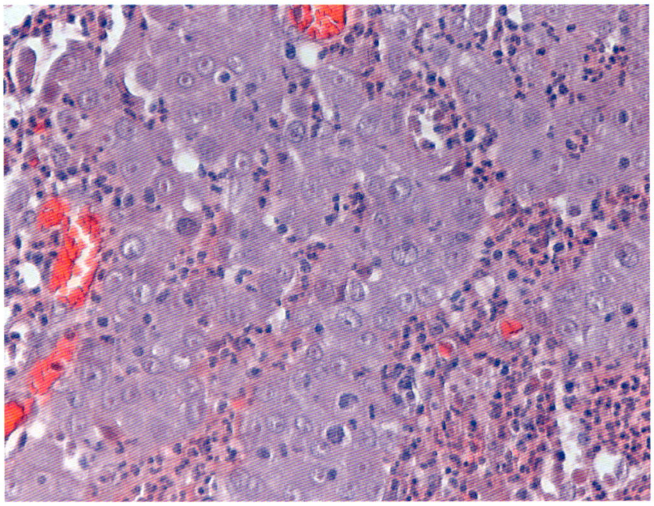

Fig. 5.16. Glassy cell carcinoma presents sheets of large cells, with a ground-glass cytoplasm and scanty intervening stroma with a prominent eosinophilic and plasma cell infiltrate.

glandular differentiation may be present [17]. Usually non-preinvasive lesions are seen (fig. 5.16).

Cytology. Cells are arranged in syncytial-like aggregates, sheets and clusters. The cells have abundant, finely granular cytoplasm ('ground-glass appearance') and large nuclei with macronucleoli. Mitoses may be numerous. Tumor diathesis, eosinophils and a lymphoplasmacytic infiltrate are usually prominent (fig. 5.17).

Diagnosis. In typical cases the smears are highly suggestive of GCC. HPV_{16} and HPV_{18} have been demonstrated in these tumors. In difficult or non-specific cases we need immunocytochemistry. The cells express cytokeratine, CEA and vimentin. HMB 45 is negative [14].

Differential Diagnosis. Atypical reparative processes may show syncytial-like aggregates, an inflammatory background and cells with prominent nucleoli, but evident malignant features are not found. Malignant tumors such as poorly differentiated non-keratinizing SCC, lymphoepithelioma-like carcinoma, metastatic carcinoma and melanoma should also be excluded.

5.4.3. Adenoid Cystic Carcinoma of the Cervix

Adenoid cystic carcinoma of the cervix resembles the salivary gland tumor of the same name, but shows greater nuclear pleomorphism, a high mitotic rate and necrosis. The majority of patients are over 60 years of age and present with bleeding and a mass on pelvic examination.

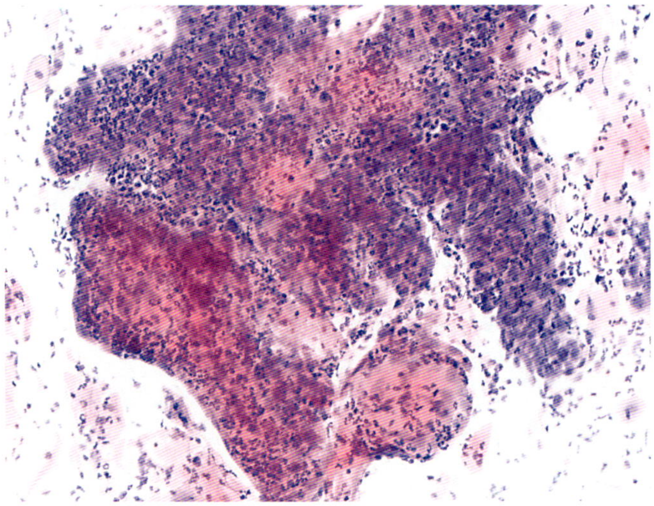

Fig. 5.17. Glassy cell carcinoma shows cells with a characteristic 'ground-glass appearance' and prominent eosinophilic and lymphoplasmacytic infiltrate.

Histology. Cystic spaces are filled with a slightly eosinophilic hyaline material or basophilic mucin and surrounded by palisaded epithelial cells.

Cytology. The cells are small and round, with dark nuclei and scant cytoplasm without mucin. They often form cell balls, which may contain hyaline globules.

Differential Diagnosis. The small size of the cells can cause confusion with benign or malignant endometrial cells. Cervical adenocarcinoma, small-cell carcinoma, poorly

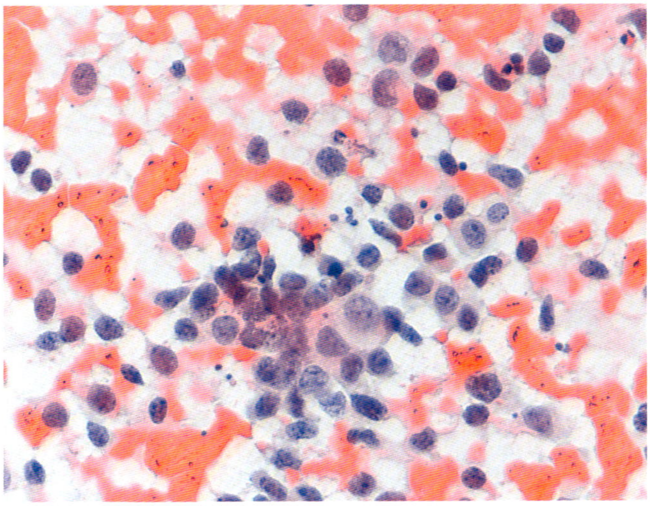

Fig. 5.18. Small round cells with scant cytoplasm and salt and pepper nuclei are characteristic of neuroendocrine tumors.

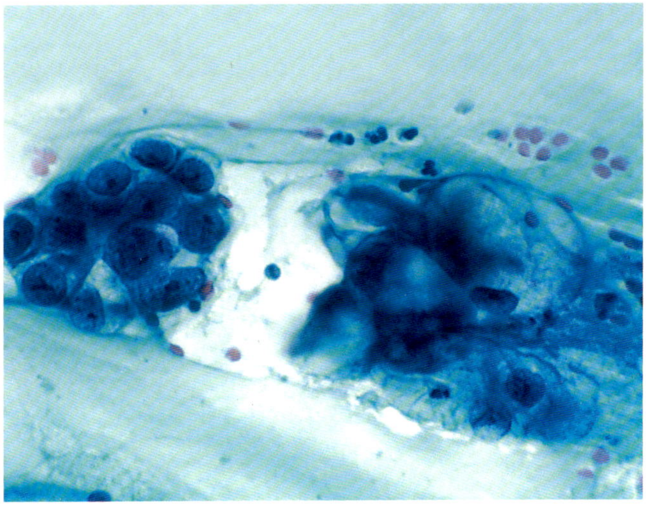

Fig. 5.19. The ovary is the most frequent origin of intragenital metastasis to the cervix.

differentiated SCC, squamous carcinoma in situ and basaloid carcinoma can also resemble adenoid cystic carcinoma.

5.4.4. Adenoid Basal Carcinoma of the Cervix

Adenoid basal carcinoma is a rare cervical carcinoma in which rounded, generally well differentiated nests of basaloid cells show focal gland formation or sometimes central squamous differentiation. The patients are generally more than 50 years old and the tumor is often discovered as an incidental finding.

Histology. Small nests of basaloid cells, almost always beneath and often arising from SIL or small invasive SCCs.

Cytology. The tumor cells form hyperchromatic crowded groups that may have peripheral nuclear palisading and a tendency to acinar formation. The cells are small, bland and uniform, with few mitotic figures. A specific diagnosis is usually not possible, except in retrospect. The associated SIL cells are generally identified.

5.4.5. Neuroendocrine Tumors

Neuroendocrine tumors include carcinoid, atypical carcinoid, large-cell neuroendocrine carcinoma and small-cell carcinoma. Neuroendocrine differentiation is demonstrated by positive staining for chromogranin A, synaptophysin and neuron specific enolase.

Generally benign carcinoids have the same characteristic organoid appearance as observed in other sites. The degree of nuclear atypia and mitotic activity is important in the differential diagnosis between typical and atypical carcinoids.

Cytology. Cellular loose aggregates or isolated small round cells with high N/C ratio, scant cytoplasm, salt-and-pepper hyperchromatic nuclei and tumor diathesis (fig. 5.18) [2, 23].

5.5. Tumors Metastatic to the Cervix

Carcinoma metastatic to the cervix is very unusual. The ovary is the most frequent origin of intragenital metastasis to the cervix (fig. 5.19) and breast and stomach are the most frequent extragenital origin. Clinical appearance of the metastatic tumors can precede diagnosis of the corresponding primary. Taking this into consideration prevents diagnostic and therapeutic errors. See chapter 11 for more details.

References

1 Atlas I, Gajewski W, Falkenberry S, Granai CO, Steinhoff MM: Absence of estrogen and progesterone receptors in glassy cell carcinoma of the cervix. Obstet Gynecol 1998;91:136–138.
2 Albores-Saavedra J: Carcinoid tumor of the uterine cervix. Virchows Arch 1984;402:331–336.
3 Ansari-Lari MA, Staebler A, Zaino RJ, Shah K, Ronnett BM: Distinction of endocervical and endometrial adenocarcinoma: immunohistochemical p16 expression correlated with human papillomavirus (HPV) DNA detection. Am J Surg Pathol 2004;28:160–167.
4 Ayer B, Pacey F, Greenberg M: The cytologic diagnosis of adenocarcinoma in situ of the cervix uteri and related lesions. II. Microinvasive Adenocarcinoma. Acta Cytol 1988;32:318–324.
5 Chang WC, Matisic JP, Zhou C, Thomson T, Clement PB, Hayes MM: Cytologic features of villoglandular adenocarcinoma of the uterine cervix: comparison with typical endocervical adenocarcinoma with a villoglandular component and papillary serous carcinoma. Cancer 1999;87:5–11.
6 Glucksmann A, Cherry CP: Incidence, histology and response to radiation of mixed carcinomas (adenoacanthomas) of the uterine cervix. Cancer 1956;9:971–979.
7 Haswani P, Arseneau J, Ferenczy A: Primary signet ring cell carcinoma of the uterine cervix: a clinicopathologic study of two cases with review of the literature. Int J Gynecol Cancer 1988;8:374–379.
8 Jiménez-Ayala M, Jiménez-Ayala Portillo B: Citopatología glandular del endocérvix: diagnóstico diferencial. Rev Esp Patol 2003;36:11–20.
9 Jones MW, Silverberg SG, Kurman RJ: Well-differentiated villoglandular adenocarcinoma of the uterine cervix: a clinicopathological study of 24 cases. Int J Gynecol Pathol 1993;12:1–7.
10 Johnson JE, Rahemtulla A: Endocervical glandular neoplasia and its mimics in ThinPrep Pap Tests: a descriptive study. Acta Cytol 1999;43:369–375.
11 Lacey JV, Brinton LA, Abbas FM, Barnes WA, Gravitt PE, Greenberg MD, Greene SM, Hadjimichael OC, Mc Gowan L, Mortel R, Mc Schwartz PE, Silverberg SG, Hildesheim A: Oral contraceptives as risk factors for cervical adenocarcinomas and squamous cell carcinomas. Cancer Epidemiol Biomarkers Prev 1999;8:1079–1085.
12 Mulvany N, Ostör A: Microinvasive adenocarcinoma of the cervix: a cytohistopathologic study of 40 cases. Diagn Cytopathol 1997;16:430–436.
13 Nevado M: Adenocarcinoma mucinoso cervical de células en anillo de sello. XVII Congreso Nacional de la SEC, Evora, 2006.
14 Reis-Filho JS, Fillus Neto J, Schonemann E, Sanderson A, Schmitt FC: Glassy cell carcinoma of the uterine cervix: report of a case with cytohistologic and immunohistochemical study. Acta Cytol 2001;45:407–410.
15 Silverberg SG, Ioffe OB: Pathology of cervical cancer. Cancer J 2003;9:335–347.
16 Solomon D, Nayar R (eds): The Bethesda System for Reporting Cervical Cytology, ed 2. New York, Springer, 2004.
17 Tavassoli FA, Devilee P: Tumors of the breast and female genital organs. WHO Classification of Tumors. Lyon, IARC Press, 2003.
18 Utsugi K, Shimizu Y, Akiyama F, Umezawa S, Hasumi K: Clinicopathologic features of villoglandular papillary adenocarcinoma of the uterine cervix. Gynecol Oncol 2004;92:64–70.
19 Vizcaino AP, Moreno V, Bosch FX, Muñoz N, Barros-Dios XM, Parkin DM: International trends in the incidence of cervical cancer. I. Adenocarcinoma and adenosquamous cell carcinoma. Int J Cancer 1988;75:536–545.
20 Young RH, Scully RE: Mucinous ovarian tumors associated with mucinous adenocarcinomas of the cervix: a clinicopathological analysis of 16 cases. Int J Gynecol Pathol 1988;7:99–111.
21 Young RH, Clement PB: Endocervical adenocarcinoma and its variants: their morphology and differential diagnosis. Histopathology 2002;41:185–207.
22 Zhou C, Gilks CB, Hayes M, Clement PB: Papillary serous carcinoma of the uterine cervix: a clinicopathologic study of 17 cases. Am J Surg Pathol 1998;22:113–120.
23 Zhou C, Hayes MM, Clement PB, Thomson TA: Small cell carcinoma of the uterine cervix: cytologyc findings in 13 cases. Cancer Cytopathol 1998;84:281–288.

Chapter 6

Endometrial Hyperplasias

6.1. Introduction

The current diagnostic strategies for the endometrial precancers are based on an integrated knowledge of endometrial carcinogenesis, from diffuse hormonal changes to benign hyperplasias and to the earliest recognizable premalignant cells (endometrial intraepithelial neoplasia, EIN) [13]. In the past, the last 2 concepts were included in the term endometrial hyperplasia (EH).

The WHO 1994 Classification System divided EH into 4 different categories based on architectural and cytological characteristics (table 6.1). Hyperplasia was designated as simple or complex (adenomatous) depending on the degree of architectural complexity, and each was subdivided into typical and atypical depending on the cytological features [5]. Recent molecular research has demonstrated that the use of the term 'hyperplasia' is conceptually correct for some but not all of these lesions. For this reason, it is currently accepted a practical classification in which the hormonal effects of unopposed estrogens (benign hyperplasia) and emergent neoplastic precancerous lesions (EIN) are separately diagnosed using non-overlapping terminology. The subset of largely polyclonal proliferations that result from a physiologic response of the endometrium to an abnormal estrogenic stimulus precisely fits the general definition of hyperplasia. In contrast, the clonal subset has the characteristics of EIN. Genetic and histological data support these 2 diagnostic terms [11].

Table 6.1. WHO Classification of endometrial hyperplasias

Typical hyperplasias
Simple hyperplasia without atypia
Complex hyperplasia without atypia (adenomatous without atypia)
Atypical Hyperplasias
Simple
Complex (adenomatous with atypia)

The diagnosis and treatment of such premalignant lesions is a major objective in the prevention of endometrial cancer and a great challenge to cytopathologists, pathologists and gynecologists [7].

6.2. Clinical Features

Benign endometrial hyperplasia occurs frequently around the time of the menopause, when both the duration and quantity of regular estrogen and progesterone production may be disturbed, but it also occurs in young women, including teenagers, in whom anovulatory cycles are also frequent [11].

The most common clinical presentation of patients with EH is abnormal uterine bleeding, whether in the form of menorrhagia, metrorrhagia or postmenopausal bleeding. Others present with abnormal vaginal discharge, or their Pap smear shows glandular abnormalities [2].

6.3. Pathophysiology

Benign endometrial hyperplasia does not have a characteristic histopathological pattern, but it rather shows sequential changes that reflect the quantity and duration of unopposed estrogen exposure. Typical histological changes include irregular remodeling of glands, sometimes accompanied by vascular thrombi, stromal breakdown and scattered cytological changes.

Prolonged estrogen exposure, unopposed by progestins, causes a modest 2- to 10-fold increase in endometrial cancer risk. Cases of benign endometrial hyperplasia that develop

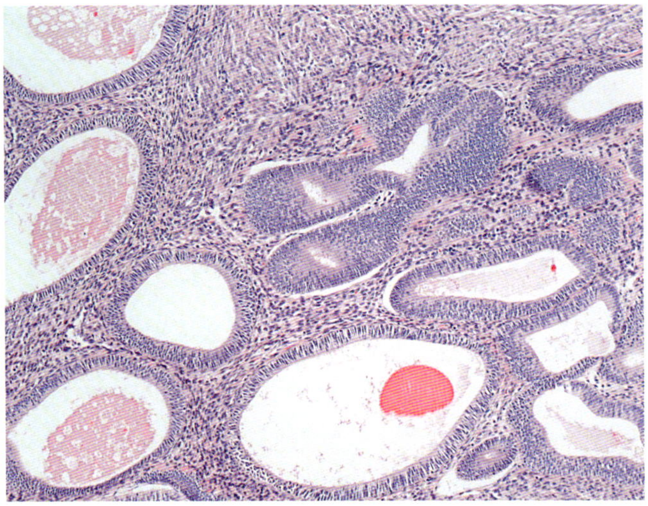

Fig. 6.1. Histology of a simple endometrial hyperplasia (WHO classification).

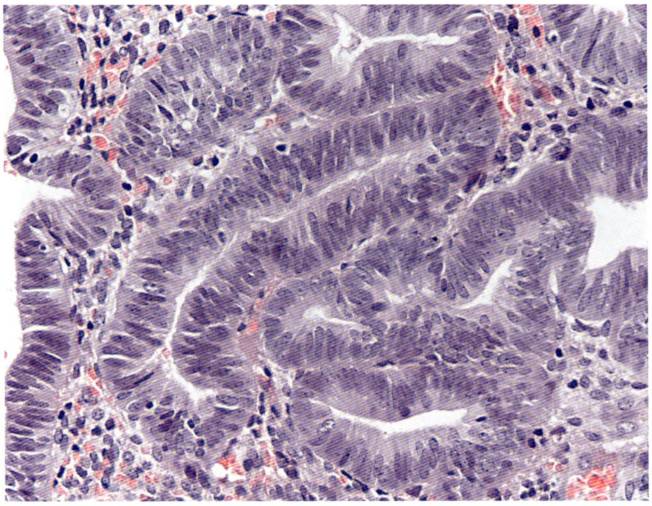

Fig. 6.2. Histology of a complex endometrial hyperplasia (WHO classification).

focal EIN are associated with a dramatically increased cancer risk [11].

Apoptosis in the glandular cells of EH is similar to the rate of apoptosis observed in proliferative endometrium. However, stromal apoptosis is decreased compared to proliferative endometrium, with a low level in all cases of EH. This decrease usually generates heavy shedding [11].

6.4. Histopathology: WHO Classification

In simple hyperplasia the endometrium is increased in volume and is qualitatively different from normal cycling endometrium. Most of the glands are rounded, but often show marked variation with cystically dilated forms. The lining epithelium is pseudostratified and lacks nuclear atypia (fig. 6.1).

Complex hyperplasia is distinguished from simple hyperplasia by a greater degree of glandular proliferation, crowding and architectural irregularity of size and shape of glands. Anarchic side buds and outpouchings explain the typical 'finger in glove' appearance. Nuclear atypia is absent (fig. 6.2).

Atypical hyperplasia (AH) affects only the glands but not the stroma. It is usually focal but may be multifocal or diffuse. The glandular epithelium presents irregular stratification and loss of nuclear polarity. The reduced stroma causes the characteristic back-to-back arrangement of the glands.

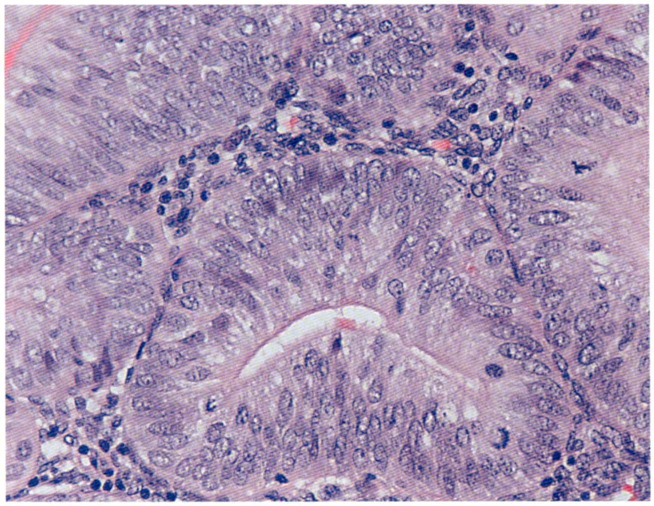

Fig. 6.3. Histology of an atypical endometrial hyperplasia (WHO classification).

The diagnostic key is the remarkable atypia of the glandular epithelial cells, both of the nuclei and of the cytoplasm, note-worthy chromatin clearing, macronucleoli, and irregular nuclear membranes [15] (fig. 6.3). Data from prospective studies have demonstrated a different risk of progression for each of the types of hyperplasia. It varies from 0 to 10% in EH without atypia to 29% in atypical complex hyperplasia [15, 16].

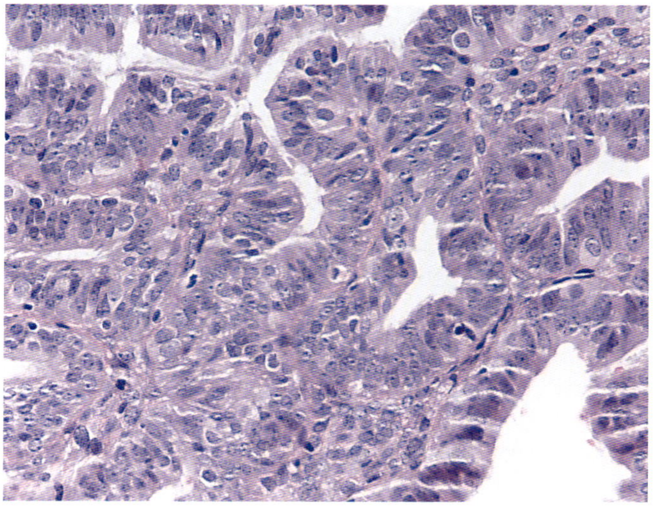

Fig. 6.4. Histology of an endometrioid neoplasia (European Pathologist Classification).

Table 6.2. Suggested European simplification of WHO Classification

WHO Classification	European Pathologist Classification 1999
Proliferative endometrium Secretory endometrium Other	Cyclical endometrium
Simple hyperplasia Complex hyperplasia	Hyperplasia
Atypical hyperplasia Well differentiated carcinoma	Endometrioid neoplasia

6.5. Multicentric European Study on Endometrial Hyperplasia

The WHO Classification of EH is generally accepted, but the assessment of cytological atypia is a key problem in assigning individual cases into 1 of the 4 different WHO categories. When we try to separate the simple and the complex categories of EH without atypia we often find overlapping histological features. A similar situation occurs in relation to the simple and complex categories of AH. Furthermore, simple AH is almost non-existent. Finally the distinction between AH and low-grade endometrial adenocarcinoma (EmA) is often difficult [1].

A multicentric European study by expert gynecological pathologists has been carried out to test the reproducibility of the WHO classification [1]. The intra-observer (85–89%) and the inter-observer (70–82%) agreements confirm that the distinction between simple and complex hyperplasia is not reproducible. Both categories have the same prognosis and the distinction is not useful to the clinician. It is preferable to assign both lesions to 1 single category, named hyperplasia. The poor agreement in the histological diagnosis of complex hyperplasia and AH, and well differentiated EmA, and the lack of reproducibility in the histological recognition of stromal alteration in differentiated AH and well differentiated EmA suggest that the WHO classification should be simplified when applied to biopsy and curettage specimens (table 6.2). This could be achieved by creating a combined category for AH and well-differentiated EmA called 'endometrioid neoplasia' (EN) (fig. 6.4). The European study found that the diagnosis of EH and EN were highly reproducible between observers from different institutions.

6.6. Diagnosis of Endometrial Hyperplasia

The diagnosis of EH is usually achieved by endometrial biopsy performed in the office, mainly using internal piston devices like the Pipelle, by dilation and curettage (D&C) or biopsy by hysteroscopy in the operating room. Tissue sampling should be carried out on women with risk factors, which present abnormal vaginal bleeding or discharge. An endometrial biopsy must be performed in all patients with cytological diagnosis of atypical glandular cells (AGC), and in women over 40 years with endometrial cells in a Pap smear [4]. Endometrial brushing techniques are a complementary tool in the investigation of this category of patients, and the method of choice to diagnose EH and early stages of EmA in women at high risk of endometrial cancer [7]. Vaginal ultrasound is also very useful in these women, as discussed in our monograph on endometrial adenocarcinoma [6].

6.7. Differential Diagnosis of Endometrial Hyperplasias

The 2 main differential diagnosis of EH are the endometrial polyp and endometrial adenocarcinoma. Endometrial polyps have some features in common with EH, but they are localized lesions with a distinctive stroma. The fibrous stroma with thick-walled blood vessels typical of polyps is not seen in benign EH (fig. 6.5) [12]. The distinction of complex hyperplasia from EmA is based on the maintained presence of stroma between the glands in complex hyperplasia and in atypical complex hyperplasia [16].

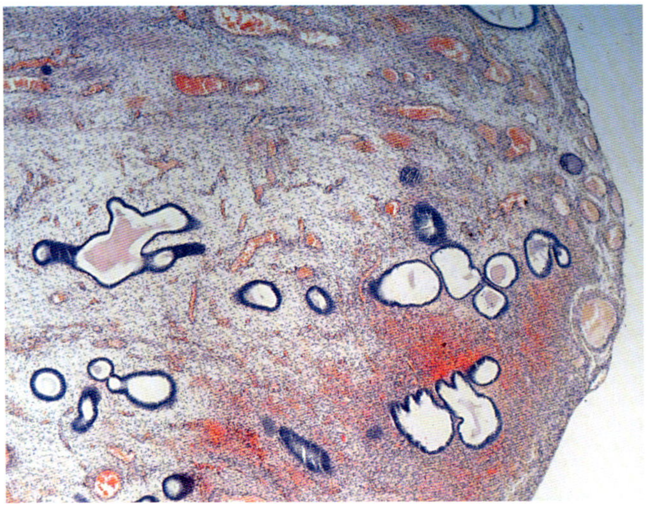

Fig. 6.5. Histology of an endometrial polyp.

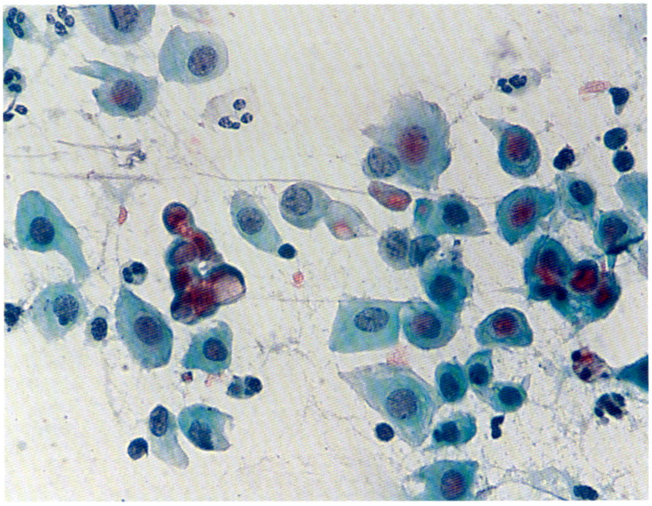

Fig. 6.6. Atypical endometrial cells in a routine Pap smear. Follow-up was a well differentiated endometrial adenocarcinoma.

6.8. Endometrial Intraepithelial Neoplasia

6.8.1. Concept

EIN is a clonal proliferation of architecturally and cytologically altered premalignant endometrial glands, which are prone to malignant transformation to endometrioid EmA (type I). EIN is not genetically invasive, it arises focally, and may transform into a malignant phenotype upon the acquisition of additional genetic damage [13].

EIN has been adopted by WHO as an alternative classification. It includes approximately 80% of the lesions which were diagnosed as complex AH in the previous system. Diagnostic criteria for EIN have been developed by histopatological correlation with clinical findings, molecular changes, and objective computerized histomorphometry [12].

6.8.2. Clinical Features

The average age at the time of EIN diagnosis is around 52 years, compared to 61 years for carcinoma. The timeframe and likelihood of EIN progression to cancer is not the same for all women. For this reason, the risk level and the management must be decided for each patient individually.

6.8.3. Diagnosis

The accepted criteria for an EIN diagnosis is a size greater than 1 mm and the cytomorphological findings of architectural crowding and a clearly abnormal background. One must exclude some lesions that can mimic cancer. The tumor suppressor gene PTEN is identified in around two thirds of all EIN lesions [13].

The importance of a correct diagnosis and treatment is obvious in view of the fact that patients with EIN lesions have an overall 89–100% increased risk of cancer compared to those without EIN [13].

6.8.4. Management of EIN

The management should be similar to that accepted for atypical endometrial hyperplasia, but we need to consider the high concurrent cancer rate (26%) and that sampling mistakes may miss a hidden tumor. This in general justifies a hysterectomy. Women with high surgical risk or women who wish to remain fertile are candidates for hormonal therapy [7]. Treatment protocols have not been standardized, but the choice depends on the severity of the lesion and on the patient's age, medical history and preferences [9].

6.9. Current Status of Cytopathology of Endometrial Hyperplasias

No specific consideration of EH is given in The Bethesda System (TBS) 2001. The only term used is AGC if all the cytological criteria for a diagnosis of glandular neoplasia are not fulfilled. AGC should be categorized as to type an origin (endocervical or endometrial; fig. 6.6). Cases of AGC may be further qualified as 'favor neoplastic'. Atypical

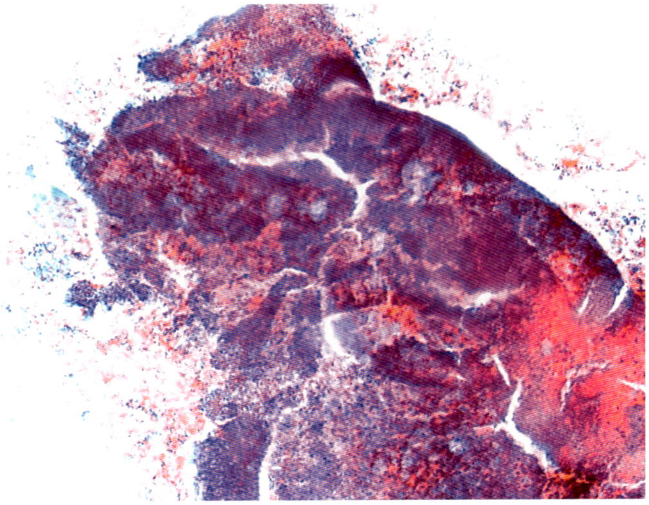

Fig. 6.7. Endometrial hyperplasia with typical abundant material (endometrial cytology).

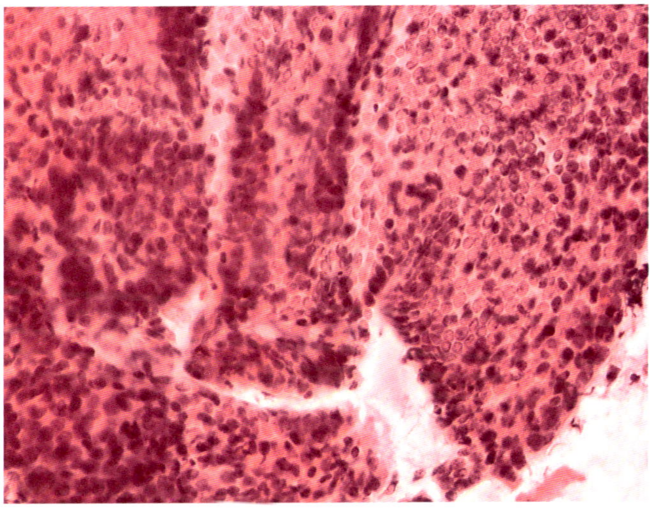

Fig. 6.8. Large sheets of endometrial cells. Endometrial hyperplasia (endometrial cytology).

endometrial cells are not further qualified due to the difficulty to subclassify this category. The cells may represent a range of histopathological lesions, such as EH, polyp or EmA [10].

The Endometrial Forum of TBS 2001 clarified that cervical cytology is primarily a screening method for squamous epithelial lesions and that it is unsuitable for the detection of endometrial lesions [17].

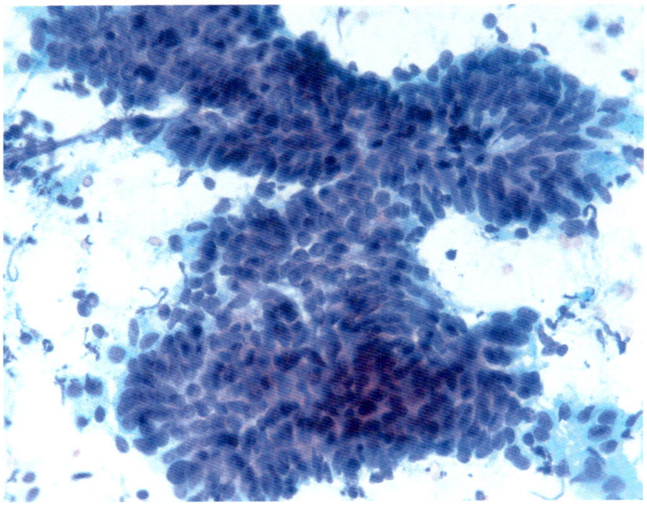

Fig. 6.9. Glandular structures. Endometrial hyperplasia (endometrial cytology).

6.10. Practical Considerations

Specific endometrial sampling techniques must be used to adequately assess the cytopathology of endometrial lesions [7]. In the interpretation of endometrial samples the cytological findings are usually combined with architectural and histological appearance [3]. Among the different methods, endometrial brushing techniques give the highest accuracy.

In 2001, after more than 35 years' experience of endometrial cytopathology, we proposed a pragmatic classification, derived from the European Pathologist Classification [8].

6.11. Cytopathology of Endometrial Hyperplasias: The Jiménez-Ayala Classification

6.11.1. Endometrial Hyperplasia (table 6.3).

We found that the simple and complex hyperplasia of the WHO Classification share the same cytopathological pattern. The material obtained by endometrial brushing techniques is abundant, showing a regular pattern of large widened glands, cell clusters and sheets of cells (fig. 6.7–6.9).

The epithelial cells are large and show slight nuclear atypia, but a uniform, finely dispersed or sometimes dense chromatin, with smooth nuclear membranes, and frequent micronucleoli. Tumor diathesis and mitotic figures are absent in the smears (fig. 6.10).

Table 6.3. Cytopathology of endometrial hyperplasia: endometrial hyperplasia. Jiménez-Ayala Classification, 2001

Arrangement	
	Regular
	Large widened glands, cell clusters and fragments
Cells	
	Somewhat large
Nuclei	
	Slight atypia, uniform
	Chromatin finely dispersed
	Smooth membrane
	Micronucleoli
Background	
	Absence of mitotic figures and tumor diathesis

Corresponding WHO classification: simple and complex hyperplasia.

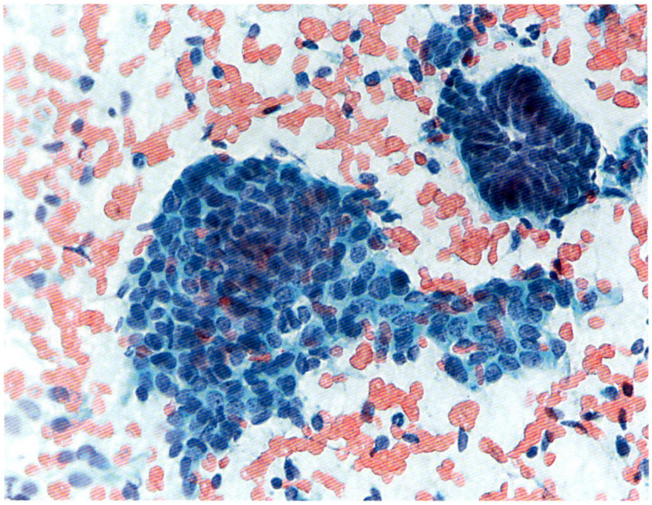

Fig. 6.10. Slight nuclear atypia with micronucleoli. Endometrial hyperplasia (endometrial cytology).

Table 6.4. Cytopathology of endometrial hyperplasia: endometrioid neoplasia. Jiménez-Ayala Classification, 2001

Arrangement	
	Large sheets
	Clusters of overlapping cells and three-dimensional groups
Cells	
	Large and pleomorphic
Nuclei	
	Large and pleomorphic
	Crowding and parachromatin clearing.
	Uneven border
	Coarse chromatin
	Nucleoli: small and medium size
Stroma	
	Large clusters
	Pale pleomorphic cells
	Oval nuclei
	Ill-defined cytoplasm
Background	
	Absent or scarce tumoral necrosis

Corresponding WHO classification: atypical hyperplasia/well differentiated adenocarcinoma.

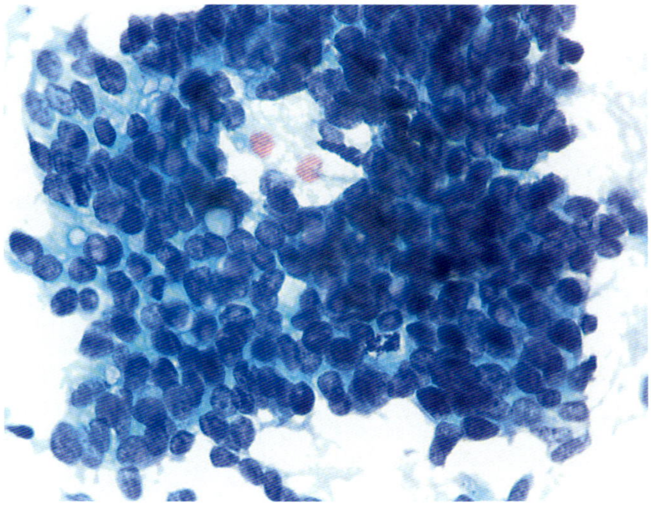

Fig. 6.11. Glandular opening, overlapping and a mitotic figure. Endometrioid neoplasia (endometrial cytology).

6.11.2. Endometrioid Neoplasia (table 6.4).

In concordance with the histopathological concept of the European Pathologist Classification, we include in this category the cytopathological feature of AH and of well-differentiated EmA. Endometrial brushing techniques show large sheets and clusters of overlapping and pleomorphic cells. The pleomorphism is, as in histologic sections, the main feature that differentiates EH from EN. The cells in 3-dimensional clusters are large with enlarged, crowded and pleomorphic nuclei. The nuclear chromatin is coarse, nuclear borders are uneven and there are small and medium-sized nucleoli contrasting with the nuclei of cells of EH (fig. 6.11–6.13). Tumoral necrosis in the smear background is absent or minimal.

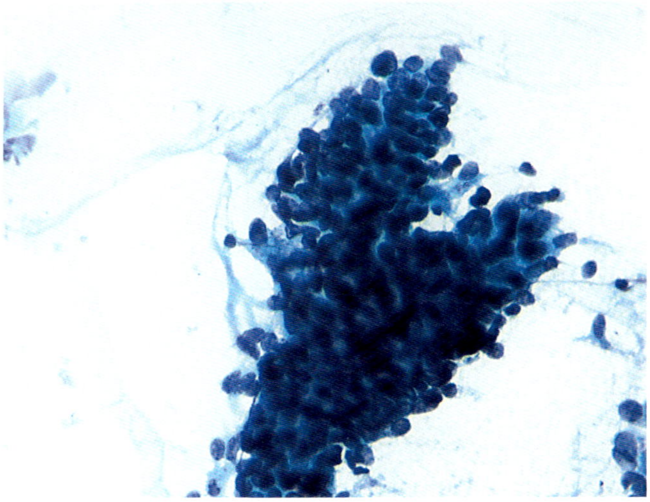

Fig. 6.12. Overlapping cells are evident in this endometrioid neoplasia (endometrial cytology).

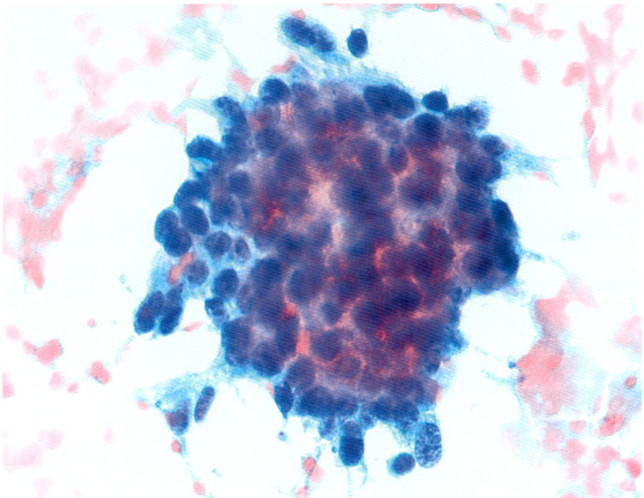

Fig. 6.13. The nuclear chromatin is coarse, and small to medium-sized nucleoli. Endometrioid neoplasia (endometrial cytology).

References

1 Bergeron C, Nogales FF, Masseroli M, Abeler V, Duvillard P, Müller-Holzner E, Pickartz H, Wells M: A multicentric European study testing the reproducibility of the WHO classification of endometrial hyperplasia with a proposal of a simplified working classification for biopsy and curettage specimens. Am J Surg Pathol 1999;23:1102–1108.

2 Chiang JW: Premalignant lesions of the endometrium, Sep 2008. E Medicine from WebMD.

3 Colgan TJ, MeLachlin M: Endometrial lesions, unusual tumors and extrauterine cancer; in Bibbo M, Wilbur DC (eds): Comprehensive cytopathology, ed 3. Amsterdam, Elsevier, 2008, pp 213–271.

4 Cowell Jl, Wilbur DC, Guidos B, Lee KR, Chhieng DC, Mody DR: Epithelial abnormalities: glandular; in Solomon D, Nayar R (eds): The Bethesda System for reporting cervical cytology, ed 2. New York, Springer 2004, pp 123–156.

5 Hecht JL, Ince TA, Baak JPA, Baker HE, Ogden MW, Mutter GL: Prediction of endometrial carcinoma by subjective endometrial intraepithelial neoplasia diagnosis. Mod Pathol 2005;18:324–330.

6 Iglesias E, Rios M: New techniques for the diagnosis of endometrial pathology, in Jiménez-Ayala M, Jiménez-Ayala Portillo B (eds): Endometrial Adenocarcinoma. Prevention and Early Diagnosis. Monogr Clin Cytol. Basel, Karger, 2008, vol 17, pp 26–31.

7 Jiménez-Ayala M, Jiménez-Ayala Portillo B (eds): Endometrial Adenocarcinoma: Prevention and Early Diagnosis. Monogr Clin Cytol. Basel, Karger, 2008, vol 17, pp 44–51.

8 Jiménez-Ayala M: Endometrial Cytology. Invited Lecture. XIV International Congress of Cytology. Amsterdam 2001.

9 Lacey JV, Ioffe OB, Ronnet BM: Endometrial carcinoma risk among women diagnosed with endometrial hyperplasia: the 34-year experience in a large health plan. Br J Cancer 2008;98:45–53.

10 Moriarty AT, Cibas ES: Endometrial cells: the how and when in reporting; in Solomon D, Nayar R (eds): Bethesda System Reporting Cervical Cytology, ed 2. New York, Springer, 2004, pp 57–66.

11 Mutter GL, The Endometrial Collaborative Group: Endometrial intraepithelial neoplasia (EIN): will it bring order to chaos? Gynecol Oncol 2000;76: 287–290.

12 Mutter GL: Histopathology of genetically defined endometrial precancers. ISGP Symposium on Endometrial Hyperplasia. Int J Gynecol Pathol 2000;19:301–309.

13 Mutter GL: Endometrial precancers: the benign endometrial hyperplasia sequence and EIN. www.endometrium.org.

14 Nguyen GK, Redburn J: Endometrial cytology by direct sampling: its value and limitations in the diagnosis of endometrial lesions; in Rosen PP, Fechner RE (eds): Pathology Annual, part 2. Stamford, Appleton and Lange, 1995, vol 30, pp 179–202.

15 Silverberg SG: Problems in the differential diagnosis of endometrial hyperplasia and carcinoma. Mod Pathol 2000;13:309–327.

16 Silverberg SG, Kurman RJ, Nogales F, Mutter GL, Kubik-Huch RA, Tavassoli FA: Epithelial tumors and related lesions; in Tavassoli FA, Devilee P (eds): Tumors of the Breast and Female Genital Organs. WHO Classification of Tumors. Lyon, IARC Press, 2003.

17 Solomon D, Nayar R (eds): The Bethesda System for Reporting Cervical Cytology, ed 2. New York Springer, 2004.

Chapter 7

Endometrial Adenocarcinoma: Current Status and Future of Prevention and Early Diagnosis

7.1. Introduction

Volume 17 of this book series was titled *Endometrial Adenocarcinoma: Prevention and Early Diagnosis* [16]. In the following chapter we summarize the most important aspects of this challenging subject and present our personal views on how to further improve the management of this important health problem.

7.2. Current Status of the Prevention and Early Diagnosis of Endometrial Adenocarcinoma

7.2.1. Increasing Incidence

Cancer has become a major public health problem in the developed world. In Europe it has a prevalence of about 3%, increasing to 5% in old age.

The results of a study published in the *European Journal of Cancer* [19] show that cancer of the uterus has an incidence of 10% and a mortality of 6%. The incidence of endometrial cancer oscillates between 9.2 (France) and 18 per 100,000 (Czech Republic). The incidence is stable in the majority of countries, except Norway, Ireland, the UK and Slovenia. In North America, endometrial cancer is the fourth most common cancer among Canadian women and represents more than 5% of all new cancer cases [6]. Most countries have experienced decreasing mortality and increasing survival rates. These recent data confirm that endometrial adenocarcinoma is the most common tumor of the female genital tract in developed countries.

7.2.2. Pathogenesis

Endometrial carcinomas are a biological and histopathological group of tumors with differing pathogenesis. The endometrioid and mucinous adenocarcinomas correspond to the estrogen-dependent carcinomas (type I; fig. 7.1). They are low-grade tumors and in most cases are associated with complex hyperplasia with cytological atypia. Serous (fig. 7.2) and clear cell carcinomas (fig. 7.3) represent high-grade tumors (type II), and they appear to be less related to sustained estrogenic stimulation. The morphologic differences in these cancers are demonstrated in their molecular genetics profile. Type I shows derangements in the PTEN gene and in the K-ras proto-oncogene. Type II is aneuploid and shows p53 mutation, also present in the precursor lesion [26].

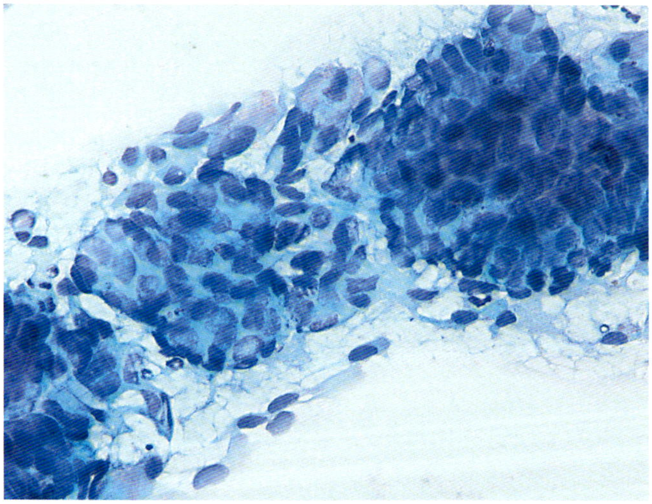

Fig. 7.1. Endometrioid adenocarcinomas correspond to estrogen-dependent carcinomas (type I).

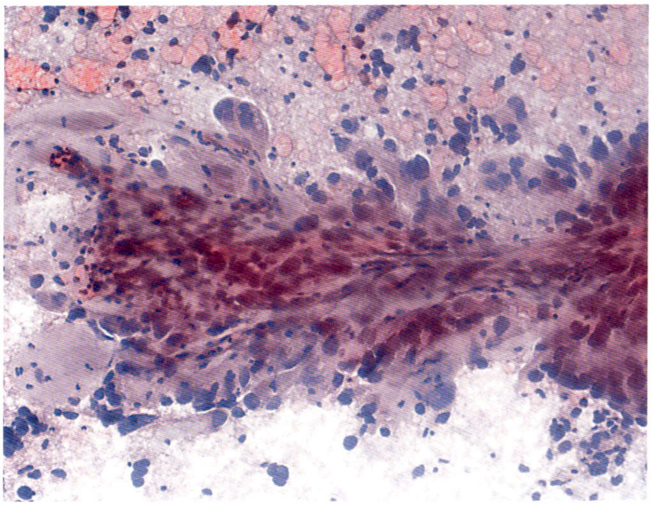

Fig. 7.2. Serous carcinomas correspond to non-estrogen-dependent carcinomas (type II).

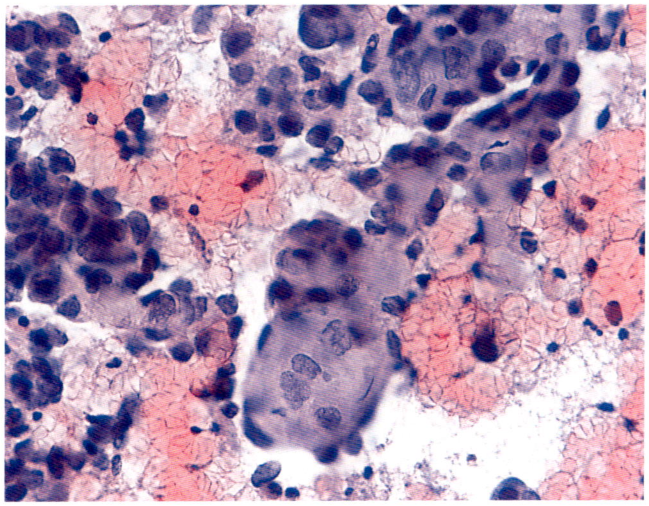

Fig. 7.3. Clear cell carcinomas are high-grade tumors (type II).

7.2.3. High-Risk Population

Epidemiological and clinical data is essential in organizing mass screening programs for the early detection of endometrial cancer.

It is important to know the prevalence of endometrial carcinomas to decide if detection is necessary and how it should be planned. Koss et al. suggested that all women over 50 should be screened at least once [20]. Grönroos et al. recommended regular mass screening programs in asymptomatic diabetic women 45 years of age or older [13].

Table 7.1. Endometrial adenocarcinoma: high-risk factors

- Estrogen-dependent adenocarcinoma (obese, diabetic, hypertensive, late menopause, multiparous); these are low-grade tumors
- Non-estrogen-dependent adenocarcinoma (older postmenopausal women); these are high-grade tumors
- Granulosa-cell tumors
- Estrogen therapy; hormone replacement treatment
- Tamoxifen

7.2.4. High-Risk Factors

High-risk factors depend on the type of endometrial adenocarcinoma (EmA). Patients with estrogen-dependent EmA (type I) are frequently obese, diabetic, multiparous, hypertensive or have a late menopause. Regarding obesity, no increase in risk factors was found in women of reproductive age, but obese postmenopausal women have a high risk of developing endometrial hyperplasia or EmA. In contrast, the non-estrogen dependent type EmA (type II) often occurs in older postmenopausal women. These women are generally not obese, diabetic or hypertensive.

Unopposed estrogen production has been shown to cause endometrial hyperplasia and EmA. This can be associated with granulosa cell tumors of the ovary or by unopposed estrogen therapy or coadjuvant therapy with tamoxifen in patients with breast cancer [1, 2]. It has been suggested that all women on tamoxifen should continue to undergo Pap tests, and that patients in whom benign endometrial cells are detected should be selected for further evaluation [12, 14] (table 7.1).

HPV does not play any role in the mutation or prognosis of EmA.

Finally, women with familiar history of hereditary nonpolyposis colorectal cancer present an increased risk of EmA.

7.2.5. Diagnostic Methods for Endometrial Screening Program

The currently most widely accepted techniques used in the detection of EmA and its precursors are:
- Cytology by endometrial brushing.
- Histopathology through office procedures: pipelle and microbiopsy.

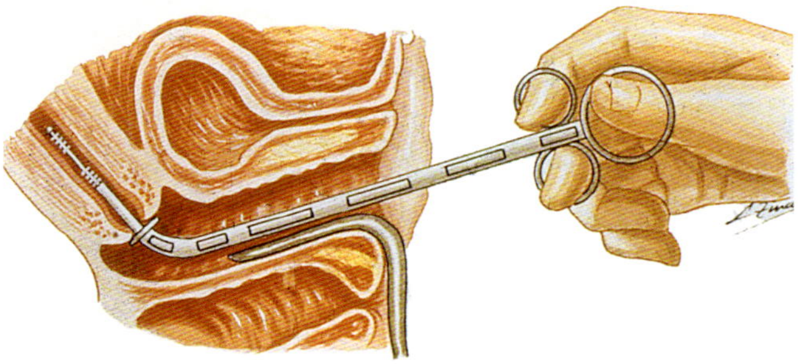

Fig. 7.4. A Medhosa cannula for endometrial brushing.

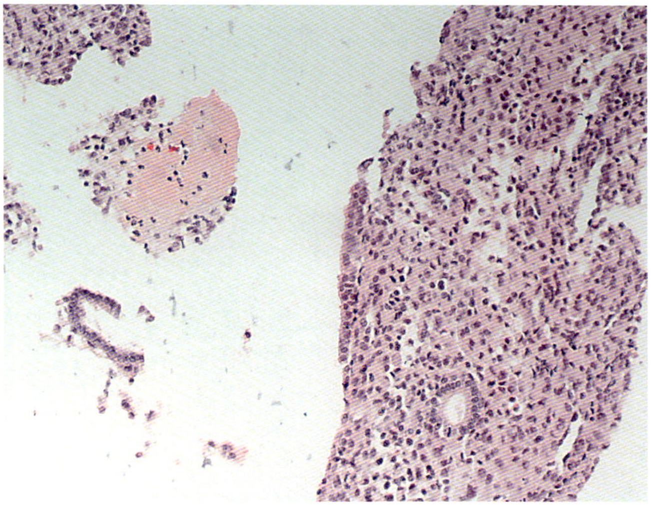

Fig. 7.6. From the same woman as in fig. 7.5. A proliferative endometrium with breakdown is seen in the cell-block preparation.

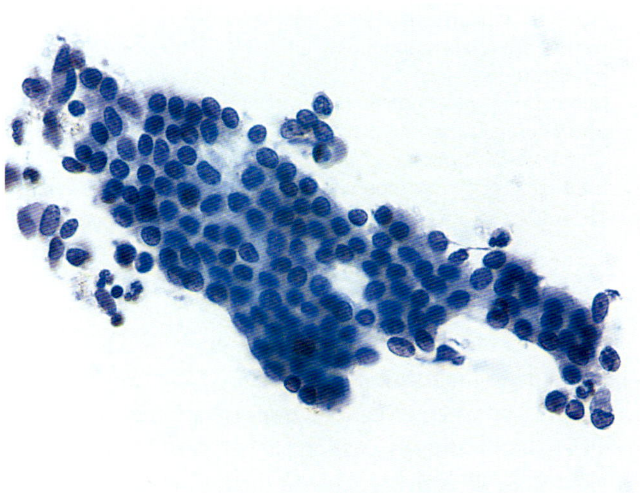

Fig. 7.5. From a 51-year-old woman with postmenopausal bleeding. Benign endometrial groups are present in the liquid-based endometrial cytology.

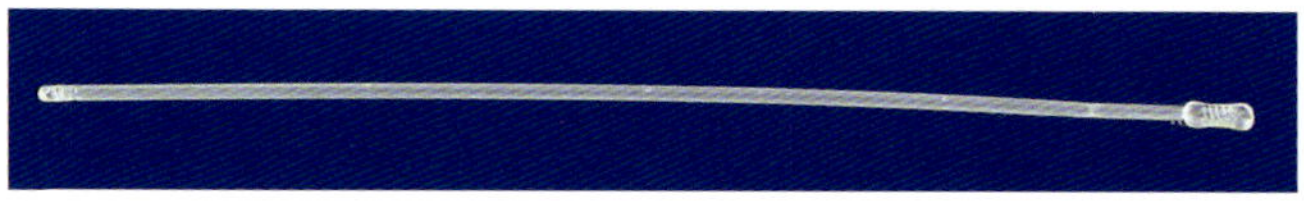

Fig. 7.7. A Pipelle, the most commonly used device for office biopsy.

- New gynecological techniques, such as transvaginal sonography and hysteroscopy.

7.2.5.1. Techniques of Endometrial Cytology

For a cytological technique to be accepted as a useful tool for endometrial screening, it must be proved to be an inexpensive, simple and painless sampling method. A second condition is that the material obtained is representative of the endometrial surface and that it permits an accurate evaluation. In a small atrophic uterus, endometrial cytology is more efficient than curettage. The endometrial brushing technique is the most commonly used sampling method for endometrial cytology [3, 23, 27, 29]. The procedures and results with different endometrial brushing techniques, and our wide experience with the Medhosa (fig. 7.4), Mi-Mark, Endobrush and Endopap methods [17, 18] were described in volume 17 of this book series [16] (table 7.2). Liquid-based endometrial cytology (fig. 7.5) [30] and cell-block preparation (fig. 7.6) were also described. These techniques have the advantage that multiple slides can be prepared for both routine and ancillary techniques, such as immunohistochemistry [9, 10, 21].

7.2.5.2. Histological Techniques

Traditionally the gold standard method for studying the endometrium and its pathology has been dilatation of the cervix and curettage under general anesthesia. It is currently accepted that histological methods for endometrial screening should be office procedures or curettage by hysteroscopy [7, 8, 22, 28, 32]. The most commonly used device for office

Table 7.2. Endometrial cytodiagnosis.

Techniques	Cases, n	Inadequate %	Correlation cyt./hist., n (%)	Adenoc., n	False positives, %	False negatives, %
Medhosa[1]	3,331	3.27	763 (22.91)	78	7.35	1.49
Endobrush[1]	404	3.00	159 (39.35)	7	0	0
Mi-Mark	8,298	12.13	1,880 (22.66)	110	3.22	1.50
Total	12,033	6.13	2,802 (28.30)	195	3.52	1.00

[1] Plus Vilaplana.

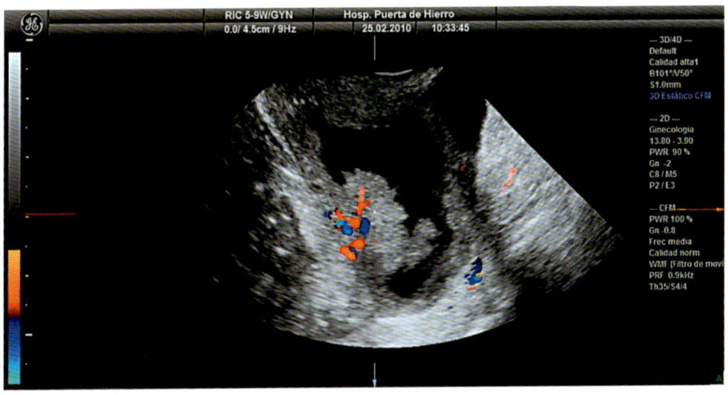

Fig. 7.8. Color-doppler of an endometrium suspected to be malignant. Newly formed endometrial vessels are seen.

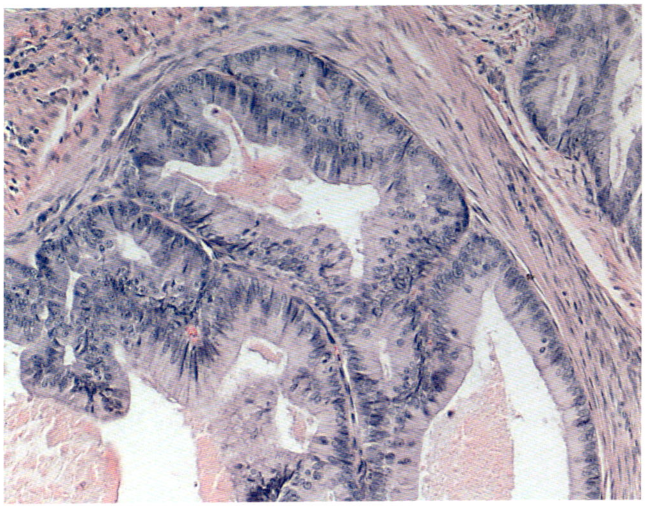

Fig. 7.9. Histology of a well differentiated endometrial adenocarcinoma (grade 1).

biopsy is the Pipelle (fig. 7.7). Both methods were presented in volume 17 of this book series [16].

7.2.5.3. New Gynecological Methods

They were presented by Enrique Iglesias and Mar Rios in the above mentioned monograph based on their wide experience with transvaginal ultrasound, including Doppler color, pulsed Doppler, 3-dimensional ultrasound and hysteroscopy in the office (fig. 7.8). Hysteroscopy-guided biopsy or curettage are probably the most accurate methods of assessing the endometrium. They permit a macroscopic evaluation of the whole uterine cavity and its pathology, providing the best result in postmenopausal women [15].

7.2.6. Histopathology of EmA: Grading

The prognostic utility of EmA grading has been recognized for many years. The most widely accepted grading system is the 1998 FIGO/ISGP with modifications suggested by Zaino et al. [33]. The WHO classification of EmA is based on architectural and nuclear features: grade 1, or well differentiated, tumors are less than 5% solid with a cribriform pattern of dilated glands, prominent nuclear atypia and mitotic activity (fig. 7.9). Grade 2, or moderately differentiated, carcinoma is 5–50% solid, the glands are smaller, with a cribriform continuous pattern (fig. 7.10). Grade 3, or poorly differentiated tumor, has an anaplastic appearance with more than 50% solid areas and few glands (fig. 7.11) [4, 31].

7.2.7. Cytopathological Grading of EmA

It is commonly accepted that for practical cytodiagnostic and prognostic purposes, EmA can cytologically be divided into 2 grades or types.

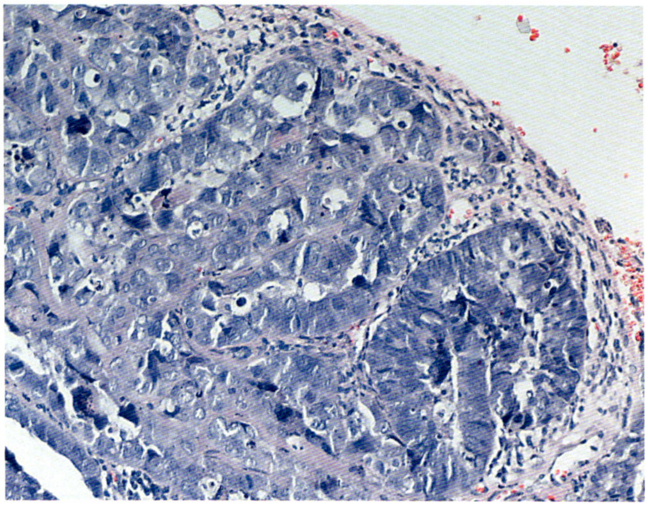

Fig. 7.10. Histology of a moderately differentiated endometrial adenocarcinoma (grade 2).

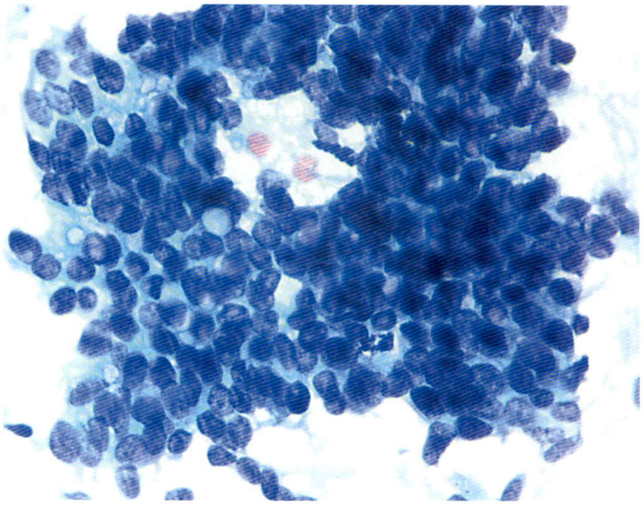

Fig. 7.12. Glandular formation and nuclear crowding in a well differentiated endometrial adenocarcinoma.

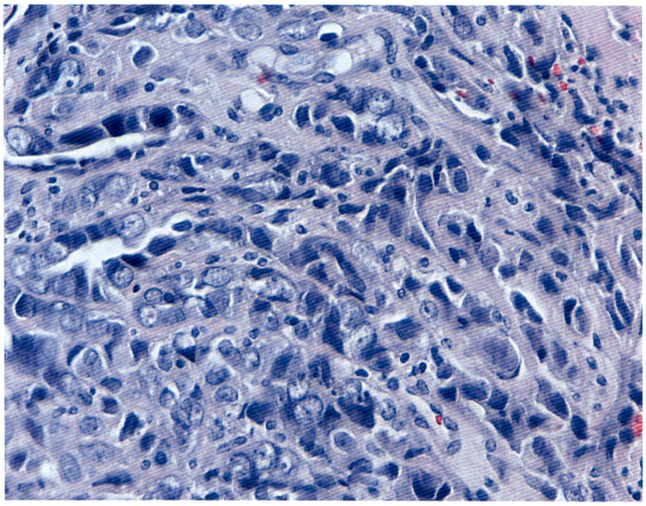

Fig. 7.11. Histology of a poorly differentiated endometrial adenocarcinoma (grade 3).

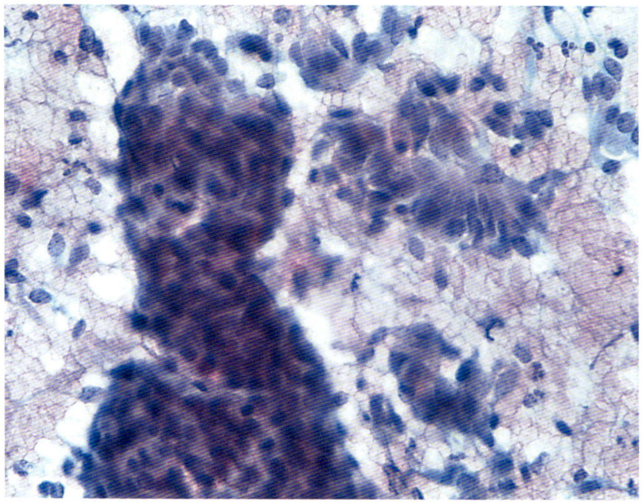

Fig. 7.13. A 3-dimensional group, aggregates of cells with pseudostratified nuclei and few isolated cells are present in this well differentiated endometrial adenocarcinoma.

7.2.7.1. Low-Grade Adenocarcinoma (Well Differentiated)

The tumor sheds in 3-dimensional, papillary structures, aggregates of cells with pseudostratified nuclei, or forms rosettes and glandular tubes. Few isolated cells are present. The cells show nuclear crowding, with anisokariosis, and usually small nucleoli. Stromal foam cells and neutrophilic emperipolesis may be present. Tumor diathesis is minimal or absent (fig. 7.12–7.14).

7.2.7.2. High-Grade Adenocarcinoma (Poorly Differentiated)

The cytologic diagnosis of high-grade adenocarcinoma is straightforward. The cells are seen as solid sheets and loose clusters, with few papillary structures. They are pleomorphic and bizarre, larger than in low grade. They show a high nuclei/cytoplasm ratio with irregular nuclear chromatin, macronucleoli and mitotic figures. Endometrial stroma is essentially absent. There is a background of necrotic debris and histiocytes (fig. 7.15).

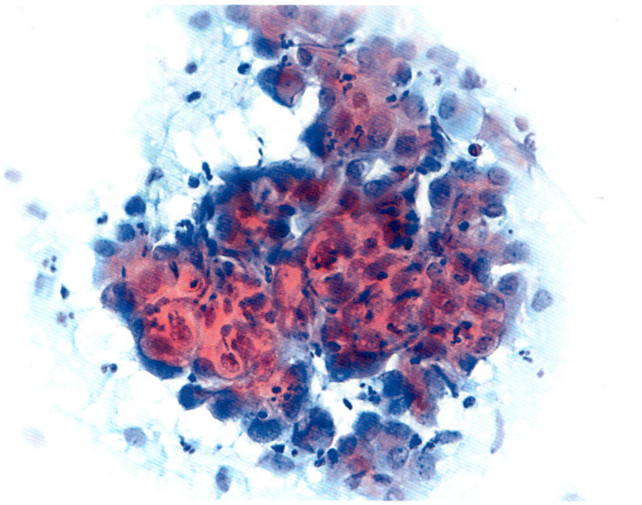

Fig. 7.14. Neutrophilic emperipolesis is typical but not specific of endometrial adenocarcinoma.

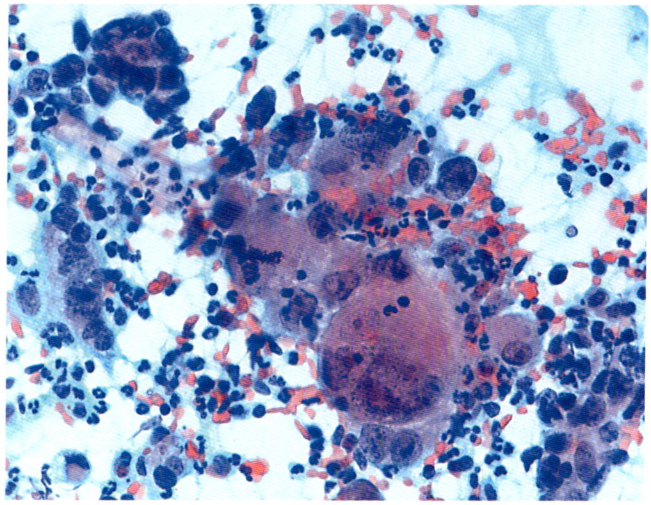

Fig. 7.15. Pleomorphic and bizarre cells with irregular nuclear chromatin, macronucleoli and atypical mitotic figures in a high-grade endometrial adenocarcinoma.

7.2.8. Liquid-Based Preparation

Tumor cells shedding from EmA appear basically similar to the counterparts in a conventional smear, but an obvious tumor diathesis is not seen due to prominent, 3-dimensional arrangements. The tumor cells are more difficult to assess. The cytoplasm is usually vacuolated or granular, and stromal histiocytes are identified [25].

7.3. Future of Prevention and Early Diagnosis

7.3.1. Challenges in Detection of Endometrial Malignant Lesions

We would like to present our personal perception based on the current knowledge of this subject and divided into the following points (table 7.3).

7.3.1.1. Assessment of High-Risk Population
In order to define the high-risk population it is necessary to plan and conduct global studies, which should include geographical distribution, race, dietary habits and age factors. As regards EmA, obesity should be a target for prevention of this growing problem [13]. It is also necessary to establish registers with uniform diagnostic and therapeutic criteria for tumor and precursor lesions in all health regions.

Table 7.3. Challenges in the detection of endometrial malignant lesions.

- Assessment of high-risk population
- Implementation of current resources
- Diagnosis and treatment of precursor lesions: hyperplasias

The CONCORD study was the first attempt to provide comparable data for cancer survival based on cancer registers in many countries [5].

An international panel of expert pathologists might help to resolve the problems of diagnostic variability between pathologists, and the differences in pathological definitions of diseases [5].

7.3.1.2. Implementation of Current Resources
In order to improve the results of the prevention and early diagnosis of EmA we need to implement the 3 most widely accepted resources, which have been mentioned above.
- Endometrial cytology should be extended to the entire high-risk population as a complementary test in the regular checking of this category of patients [27].
- Endometrial tissue pathology. These efficient methods should be used more extensively. They are easy to use when employed as an office procedure.
- New gynecological techniques for the diagnosis of endometrial pathology. Transvaginal ultrasound and

hysteroscopy-guided biopsy have been unanimously accepted and their use should also be implemented [15].

7.3.1.3. Diagnosis and Treatment of Premalignant Lesions: Hyperplasia

Primary prevention strategies aimed at reducing the risk of EmA need to initially focus on precursors. The current position of these strategies includes dealing with the above mentioned high-risk factors, and assessment of abnormal bleeding, the most frequent sign of both EmA and its precursors. Early diagnosis of these lesions is essential to achieve a more favorable prognosis [19, 24].

7.4. Conclusion

As a final conclusion, we would like to emphasize a few points. Cancer prevention and management of uterine corpus neoplasia in Europe is moving in the right direction. The combination of earlier detection and better access to cases and improved treatment have achieved increased survival rates and decreased mortality. Nevertheless, there are important challenges that we feel could be solved or at least reduced by the implementation of the strategies mentioned above. Other possible means of prevention are to dissuade women from smoking, to fight the emerging obesity epidemic [11, 19], to decrease estrogen exposure and to pay special attention to abnormal vaginal bleeding that may be the result of tumoral necrosis and breakdown in endometrial carcinoma [3, 6].

References

1 Abadi MA, Barakat RR, Saigo PE: Effects of tamoxifen on cervicovaginal smears from patients with breast cancer. Acta Cytol 2000;44:141–146.
2 Benson JR, Pitsinis V: Update on clinical role of tamoxifen. Curr Opin Obstet Gynecol 2003;15: 13–23.
3 Buratti E, Cetis F, Masserini M, Goisis F, Vergadoro F, Bolis G: The value of endometrial cytology in a high-risk population. Tumori 1985;71:25–28.
4 Clement PB, Young RH: Endometrioid carcinoma of the uterine corpus: a review of its pathology with emphasis on recent advances and problematic aspects. Adv Anat Pathol 2002;9:145–184.
5 Coleman MP, Quaresma M, Berrino F, Lutz JM, De Angelis R, Capocaccia R: Baili P, Rachet B, Gatta G, Hakulinen T, Micheli A, Sant M, Weir HK, Elwood JM, Tsukuma H, Koifman S, E Silva GA, Francisci S, Santaquilani M, Verdecchia A, Storm HH, Young JL; CONCORD Working Group: Cancer survival in five continents: a worldwide population-based study. Lancet Oncol 2008;9:730–756.
6 Colgan TJ, McLachlin CM: Endometrial lesions, unusual tumors and extrauterine cancer; in Bibbo M, Wilbur DC (eds): Comprehensive Cytopathology, ed 3. Amersterdam, Elsevier, 2008, pp 247–271.
7 Cornier E: The Pipelle: a disposable device for endometrial biopsy. Am J Obstet Gynecol 1984;148: 109–110.
8 Del Priore G, Williams R, Harbatkin CB, Wan LS, Mittal K, Yang GC: Endometrial brush biopsy for the diagnosis of endometrial cancer. J Reprod Med 2001;46:439–443.
9 De May RM: The Pap test. Chicago, ASCP Press, 2005, pp 119–152.
10 Diaz-Rosario LA, Kabawat SE: Cell block preparation by inverted filter sedimentation is useful in the differential diagnosis of atypical glandular cells of undetermined significance in the ThinPrep specimens. Cancer 2000;90:265–272.
11 Papanas N, Giatromanolaki A, Galazios G, Maltezos E, Sivridis E: Endometrial carcinoma and diabetes revisited. Eur J Gynaecol Oncol 2006;27: 505–508.
12 Greenspan DL, Cardillo M, Davey DD, Heller DS, Moriarty AT: Endometrial cells in cervical cytology: review of cytological features and clinical assessment. J Low Genit Tract Dis 2006;10:111–122.
13 Grönroos M, Salmi TA, Vuento MH, Jalava EA, Tyrkkö JE, Maatela JI, Aromaa AR, Siegberg R, Savolailen ER, Kauraniemi TV: Mass screening for endometrial cancer directed in risk groups of patients with diabetes and patients with hypertension. Cancer 1993;71:1279–1282.
14 Hachisuga T, Saito T, Kigawa J, Ohwada M, Yamazawa K, Yasue A, Iwasaka T, Sugiyama T, Kita T, Nagai N: Clinicopathologic study of 56 patients with endometrial cancer during or after adjuvant tamoxifen use of their breast cancer. Gynecol Oncol 2004;95:139–144.
15 Iglesias E, Rios M: New techniques for the diagnosis of Endometrial Pathology; in Jiménez-Ayala M, Jiménez-Ayala Portillo B (eds): Endometrial Adenocarcinoma: Prevention and Early Diagnosis. Monogr Clin Cytol. Basel, Karger, 2008, vol 17, pp 26–31.
16 Jiménez-Ayala M, Jiménez-Ayala Portillo B (eds): Endometrial Adenocarcinoma: Prevention and Early Diagnosis. Monogr Clin Cytol. Basel, Karger, 2008, vol 17.
17 Jiménez-Ayala M, Vilaplana E, Becerro de Bengoa C, Zomeño M, Moreno S, Granados M: Endometrial and endocervical brushing techniques with a Medhosa cannula. Acta Cytol 1975; 19:557–563.
18 Jiménez-Ayala M: Endometrial cytology: yesterday, today, tomorrow. Goldblatt Lecture. XII International Congress of Cytology, Madrid, 1995.
19 Karim-Kos HE, De Vries E, Soerjomataram I, Lemmens V, Siesling S, Coebergh JW: Recent trends of cancer in Europe: a combined approach of incidence, survival and mortality for 17 cancer sites since the 1990s. Eur J Cancer 2008;44: 1345–1389.
20 Koss LG, Schreiber K, Oberlander SG, Moussouris HF, Lesser M: Detection of endometrial carcinoma and hyperplasia in asymptomatic women. Obstet Gynecol 1984;64:1–11.
21 Kyroudi A, Paefthimiou M, Symiakaki H, Mentzelopoulou P, Voulgaris Z, Karakitsos P: Increasing diagnostic accuracy with a cell-block preparation from thin-layer endometrial cytology: a feasibility study. Acta Cytol 2006;50:63–69.
22 Machado F, Moreno J, Carazo M, Leon J, Fiol G, Serna F: Accuracy of endometrial biopsy with the Cornier pipelle for the diagnosis of endometrial cancer and atypical hyperplasia. Eur J Gynaecol Oncol 2003;24:279–281.
23 Meissels A, Morin C: Modern Uterine Cytopathology. Chicago, ASCP Press, 2007.
24 Mencaglia J, Valle RF, Perino A, Gilardi G: Endometrial carcinoma and its precursors: early detection and treatment. Int J Gynaecol Obstet 1990;31:107–116.
25 Mody DR: Glandular lesions in cervicovaginal cytology: conventional, ThinPrep and SurePath. Microscopic Tutorial 10. 53rd Annual Scientific Meeting of the American Society of Cytopathology. San Diego, 2005, pp 1–15.

26 Mutter GL: Histopathology of genetically defined endometrial precancers. ISGP Symposium on Endometrial Hyperplasia. Int J Gynecol Pathol 2000;19:301–309.
27 Nguyen GK, Redburn J: Endometrial cytology by direct sampling: its value and limitations in the diagnosis of endometrial lesions. Pathol Annu 1995; 30:179–202.
28 Ono M, Shiina Y, Sakuma K, Inoue H: Method of producing tissue sections from endometrial scrapings. Cytopathology 2002;13:46–53.
29 Palermo VG: Interpretation of endometrium obtained by Endopap sampler and a clinic study of its use. Diagn Cytopathol 1985;1:5–12.
30 Papaefthimiou M, Symiakaki H, Mentzelopoulou R, Giahnaki AE, Voulgaris Z, Diakomanolis E, Jyroudes A, Karakitsos P: The role of liquid-based cytology associated with curettage in the investigations of endometrial lesions from postmenopausal women. Cytopathology 2005;16:32–39.
31 Silverberg SG, Kurtman RJ, Nogales F, Mutter GL, Kubik-Huch RA, Travassoli FA: Epithelial tumors and related lesions; in Tavassoli FA, Devilee P (eds): Tumors of the Breast and Female Genital Organs: WHO Classification of Tumors. Lyon, IARC Press, 2003.
32 Wu HH, Casto BD, Elsheikh TM: Endometrial brush biopsy: an accurate outpatient method of detecting endometrial malignancy. J Reprod Med 2003;48:41–45.
33 Zaino RJ, Kurtman RJ, Diana KL, Morrow CP: The utility of the revised International Federation of Gynecology and Obstetric histologic grading of endometrial adenocarcinoma using a defined nuclear grading system. A Gynecology Oncology Group Study. Cancer 1995;75:81–86.

Chapter 8

Cytopathology of Ovarian Lesions: The Intraoperative Approach

8.1. Introduction

The study of cytological specimens as a complementary tool to frozen sections in the intraoperative consultation for ovarian lesions improves the performance of intraoperative diagnosis. Although cytology imprints and smears have been used by pathologists for many years as an adjunct to frozen sections in various organs, this has not been the case for the ovary. The increasing demand for intraoperative procedures in the diagnosis of ovarian tumors makes us aware of the importance of including diagnosis of cytological specimens in the study of frozen sections [10, 15, 22, 26].

The reliability of intraoperative consultation for ovarian tumors has been highlighted by many authors, who report a high percentage of concordance and overall accuracy between frozen sections and definitive paraffin sections, with values ranging from 87 to 96% [1–3, 7–9, 16, 19, 26]. Few studies have provided information regarding the improved performance obtained by adding cytology to frozen sections in the intraoperative procedure. Cytology is a simple and rapid technique that provides high quality diagnostic specimens. Cytological specimens can overcome some of the diagnostic limitations of frozen sections.

Rapid intraoperative diagnosis relies on macroscopic examination, frozen sections and, in our experience, they also depend on cytology and cytopathologic correlation.

Pathologic features of ovarian lesions described by several authors are summarized [4, 13, 17, 18, 24, 27].

Intraoperative cytomorphology of ovarian tumors is described using information obtained from the intraoperative pathology records of our laboratory. During the period from January 2005 to May 2009, 337 cases of intraoperative consultations for ovarian neoplastic and non-neoplastic lesions were carried out, accounting for 14% of a total of 2,327 ovarian lesions analyzed during that period.

Reference textbooks describe cytomorphologic features of ovarian lesions in specimens obtained by fine needle aspiration [5, 6, 12].

8.2. Histology and Cytology of Ovarian Lesions

8.2.1. Epithelial-Stromal Ovarian Tumors

This category accounts for two thirds of all ovarian tumors, and 90% of all ovarian malignant tumors. They are subclassified based on the epithelial component as serous, mucinous, clear cell, endometrioid and transitional, with benign, borderline and malignant variants. This latter division is done according to the amount of tumor cell proliferation, nuclear atypia and the presence or absence of stromal invasion. Borderline tumors, by definition, show epithelial proliferation greater than that seen in benign tumors, and they do not exhibit destructive invasion of the stroma.

It must be underscored that the gross appearance of the different subtypes of epithelial tumors have frequent common features, presenting as cystic, uni- or multilocular morphology, with focal or diffuse papillary and polypoid projections and excrescences lining the internal and/or external surfaces. Fluid contents may be clear, serous, mucinous or hemorrhagic, and they are non-specific to any of the histological subtypes. These macroscopic manifestations are shared by borderline and malignant epithelial tumor variants. Benign follicular, functional and endometriotic cysts may present as cystic tumors with somewhat irregular inner surfaces and similar fluid contents. Some of the gross features of solid tumors with multinodular, necrotic and hemorrhagic areas are shared by primary and metastatic tumors.

The heterogeneity of the macroscopic presentation determines the need for extensive sampling, which cannot be fully performed during intraoperative consultation. Deferring to definitive diagnosis in paraffin sections must be considered.

These shared gross features give frozen sections and cytological specimens the status of important diagnostic adjunctive methods that help determine further surgical management and staging.

8.2.1.1. Serous Carcinomas

Serous carcinomas are 20–25% of the serous ovarian tumors. The mean age of presentation is 56 years; 70% of the cases are diagnosed in an advanced stage with extra-ovarian dissemination. The epithelial component with cylindrical ciliated cells resembles the epithelium that lines the fallopian tube.

Macroscopy. Two thirds of the cases are bilateral, and their diameters range from microscopic to ≥20 cm. Well-differentiated serous carcinomas are solid/cystic masses with soft and friable papillary projections lining the inner surface focally or diffusely. Papillary projections may also be present on the external surface. Exophytic and intracystic endophytic gross presentation may occur simultaneously or independently. Poorly differentiated serous tumors are usually multinodular and solid, with areas of necrosis and hemorrhage.

Microscopy. These tumors are usually high grade, and they typically show a complex papillary pattern with marked, irregular branching of the epithelial proliferation, with very scarce or no stromal support. There are obvious signs of stromal invasion. Cells may be small and medium-sized, with a few sparse multinucleated, bizarre giant cells. Numerous mitoses may be found. Solid cellular proliferation, small acini and longitudinal slit-like spaces can be observed in a scanty and desmoplastic stroma. Necrosis may be prominent and psammoma bodies are typically found in these tumors.

Low-grade, well-differentiated tumors are less frequent. Usually they show a papillary pattern with prominent fibrous cores and obvious stromal invasion by single cells and small epithelial nests.

Differential Diagnosis. Primary serous tumor of the peritoneum, endometrioid, clear cell and transitional cell carcinomas with a papillary pattern, malignant mesothelioma, metastatic serous carcinoma of tubes and endometrium, metastatic breast tumors.

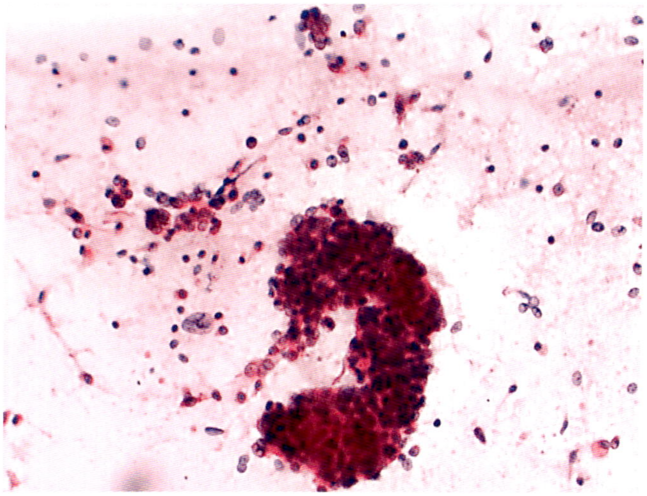

Fig. 8.1. Serous papillary carcinoma. Dense papillary clusters, loose aggregates of epithelial cells with loss of polarity and cohesiveness and single cells. Variation in size and shape of nuclei, hyperchromasia, irregular chromatin and prominent nucleoli. HE, 10×.

Cytology. Cytological specimens show high cellularity. There are numerous 3-dimensional dense cell papillary clusters and loose aggregates of abnormal epithelial cells with loss of polarity and cohesiveness, as well as single cells and bizarre cells. Cells have small amounts of granular cytoplasm, with occasional vacuoles. Nuclei show variations in size and shape, hyperchromasia and moderate-to-high nuclear atypia with high N/C ratios. Nuclei have granular or coarse clumped chromatin that is irregularly distributed. Both prominent nucleoli and macronucleoli are frequent findings, and psammoma bodies may also be found occasionally. The tumor background tends to be hemorrhagic and necrotic. A marked nuclear pleomorphism is typically apparent in poorly differentiated serous carcinomas (fig. 8.1–8.3).

8.2.1.2. Psammomacarcinoma

Psammomacarcinomas are very rare tumors that correspond to low-grade serous carcinomas. The histological pattern shows papillae and epithelial nests invading a fibrous stroma. Low-to-moderate nuclear atypia is usual. Psammoma bodies are seen in 75% or more of the epithelial component.

Cytology. Cytological specimens show high cellularity, with numerous single cells and 3-dimensional epithelial aggregates and papillae. Nuclei are round to ovoid in

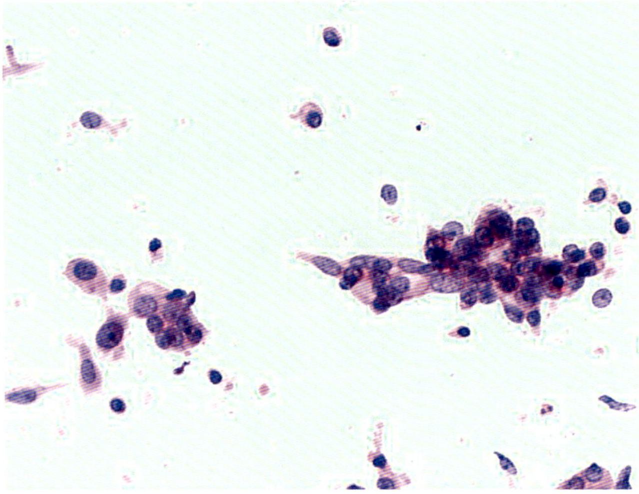

Fig. 8.2. Serous papillary carcinoma. Loose aggregates of apithelial cells, small acini. Three-dimensional dense, papillary groups. Loss of polarity and cohesiveness. Anisonucleosis, irregular chromatin, prominent nucleoli, scanty cytoplasm. HE, 20×.

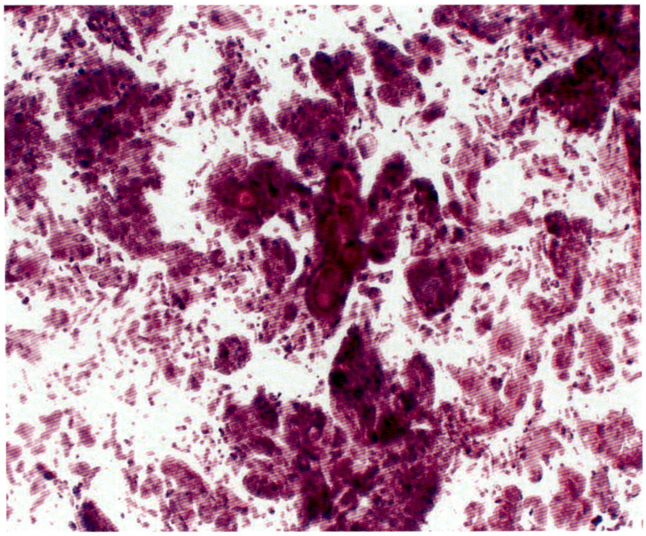

Fig. 8.4. Psammomacarcinoma. High cellularity. Three-dimensional epithelial aggregates, papillae and single cells. Numerous psammoma bodies lying over the epithelial component or free in the background. HE, 10×.

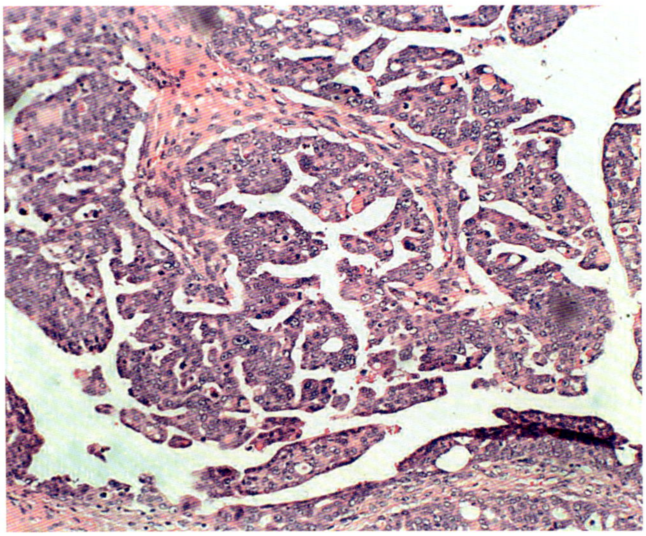

Fig. 8.3. Serous papillary carcinoma. Complex papillary pattern with irregular branching of closely packed papillae. Atypical nuclei, high N/C ratio, prominent nucleoli. HE, 10×.

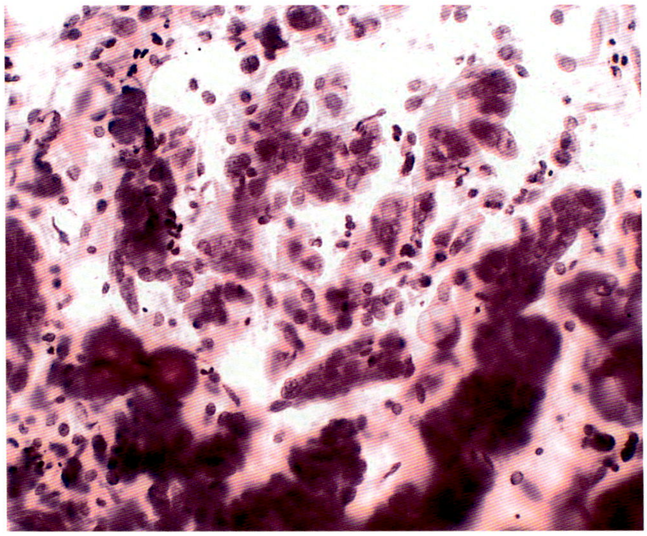

Fig. 8.5. Psammomacarcinoma. Epithelial cells with round or vesicular nuclei, granular and fine or irregular, coarse chromatin, distinct nucleoli. Psammoma bodies. HE, 20×.

shape, and slightly hyperchromatic or vesicular and clear. Chromatin may be granular or clumped, and nucleoli are fine or prominent. The presence of numerous psammoma bodies associated to the epithelial component or lying free in the background is a typical finding (fig. 8.4–8.6).

8.2.1.3. Serous Borderline Tumors

Serous borderline tumors (SBT) represent 10% of the serous tumors of the ovary. They occur 10 years earlier than serous carcinomas, at a mean age of 42 years. They are rare in women under 20 years of age; 30% of the patients have bilateral tumors. Seventy percent of the cases are diagnosed in stage I, having a favorable prognosis.

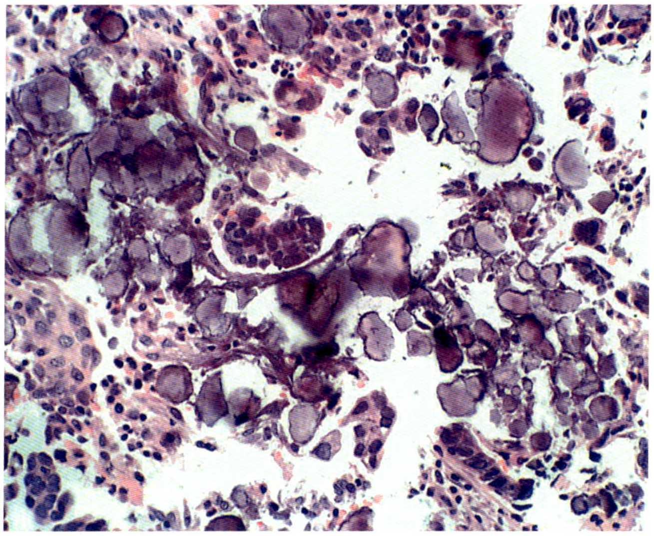

Fig. 8.6. Psammomacarcinoma. Epithelial papillae and nests. Multiple psammoma bodies. Stromal invasion. Low to moderate atypia. Paraffin section. HE, 20×.

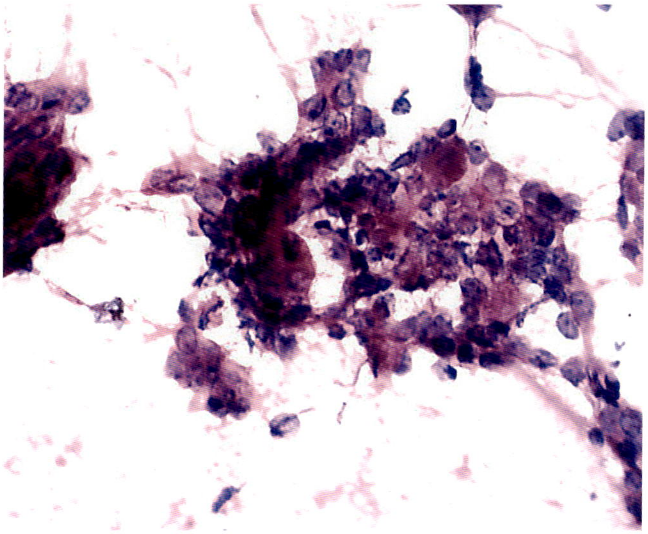

Fig. 8.7. Serous borderline tumor. Two- and three-dimensional dense cell aggregates with irregular contours. Loss of polarity and cohesivity. HE, 20×.

When a borderline tumor is suspected during the intraoperative consultation, definitive paraffin sections may be necessary to rule out invasion.

Macroscopy. The gross examination shows cystic, mono- or multiloculated tumors. The inner surface is focally or totally lined by papillary and polypoid excrescences of variable diameters, usually firm and white. Although it is possible to see an exclusive superficial exophytic gross presentation, it is usually associated with an endophytic component. There is typically no necrosis or hemorrhage.

Microscopy. Two histological variants of borderline serous tumors are described. (a) Typical or common SBT shows a hierarchical complex papillary pattern, without stromal invasion. Papillae show a stratified cuboidal-columnar epithelium with abundant fibrous cores. Cells have low nuclear atypia, slight hyperchromasia and scarce mitosis. (b) Micropapillary SBT shows a complex, irregular and non-hierarchical papillary pattern that must measure more than 5 mm in linear extension. Cribriform areas may also be associated. The papillae consist of stratified cuboidal-columnar epithelium with a high N/C ratio. Detachment of the apical epithelial nests of the papillae into the cystic lumen is typical. Nuclear atypia is low to moderate, with fine nucleoli and mitosis are rare. Areas of typical SBT patterns are usually associated. One or more foci of stromal micro-invasion are present in 10% of the SBT. Images of stromal micro-invasion consist of the presence of single cells, nests, papillae and acini, some of them with cells showing an abundant eosinophilic cytoplasm, which may be surrounded by clear spaces. Arbitrarily, these foci must not exceed 10 mm^2, or 3 mm in maximal linear extension.

Differential Diagnosis. Serous carcinoma, mucinous borderline endocervical-like tumor, retiform Sertoli-Leydig cell tumors.

Cytology. Cytological specimens show 2 or 3-dimensional dense cellular groups with irregular contours and papillary configuration. Cell aggregates show slight loss of polarity and cohesiveness. Small solid epithelial nests may be seen protruding, detached and shed into the lumen at the periphery of the cellular groups and they may correspond to the apical epithelial nests seen in histology. These epithelial nests may be seen lying free in the background near the papillary groups. There are typically very few isolated cells. Most commonly the cells show uniform, bland nuclei with low to moderate atypia. Delicate granular chromatin, regularly distributed and fine or inconspicuous nucleoli is seen. Mitosis are infrequent. Psammoma bodies may be found.

A benign component is usually identified, showing single cylindrical, sometimes ciliated cells and papillary cohesive 2- or 3-dimensional clusters. Ovoid bland nuclei, with no nuclear atypia are found (fig. 8.7–8.9).

8.2.1.4. Mucinous Carcinoma

The frequency of primary ovarian mucinous adenocarcinoma (MA) has dropped from the reported 15% to almost 3%, because of several factors, such as the acceptance of a

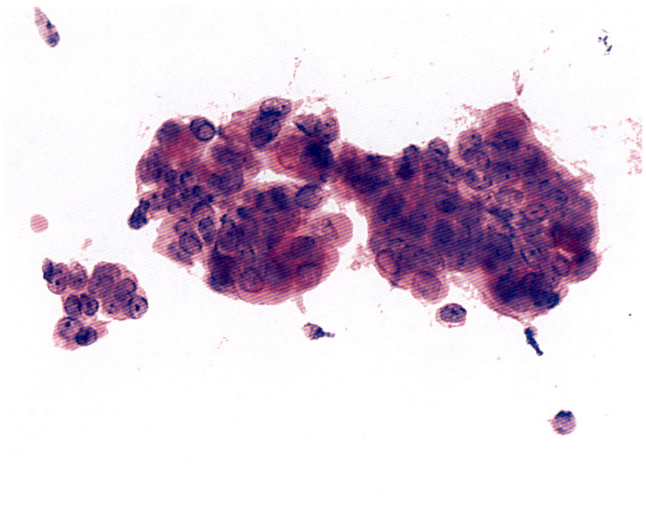

Fig. 8.8. Serous borderline tumor. Papillary group with peripheral detachment of small epithelial nests. Low to moderate nuclear atypia, scarse prominent nucleoli. HE, 20×.

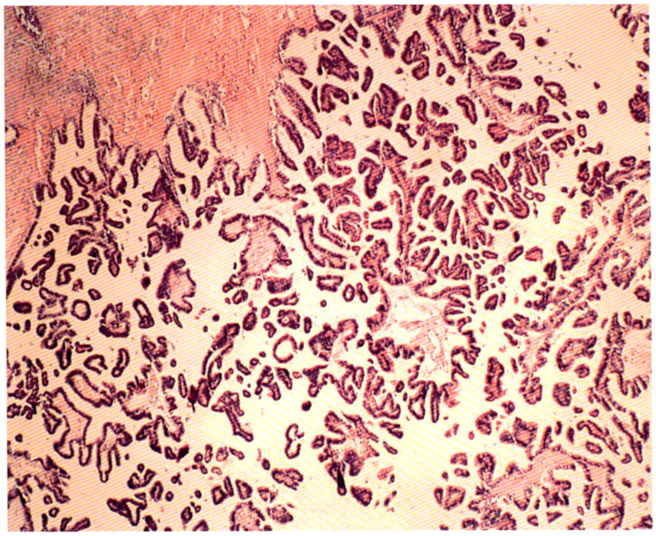

Fig. 8.9. Serous borderline tumor, typical pattern. Hierarchical and complex papillary pattern. No stromal invasion. HE, 20×.

borderline mucinous tumor category, the confirmation of the existence of metastatic mucinous tumors that resemble primary MA, and recognition that mucinous tumors with pseudomyxoma peritonei are actually metastases originating from the appendix.

Macroscopy. The typical primary MA is a unilateral tumor involving only 1 ovary (stage I). These tumors are large, cystic, multiloculated masses with papillary and solid areas. A mucinous content and areas of necrosis and hemorrhage are usually found. Integrity of the capsule must always be assessed.

Microscopy. Two variants of MA are identified histologically, depending on the patterns of their stromal invasion: typical infiltrative invasion and expansile-type invasion. Typical infiltrative invasion shows desmoplastic stroma with disorderly invasion by irregular glands, individual epithelial cells or groups of cells with abundant cytoplasm, some of which are surrounded by clear spaces. The expansile type has no demonstrable destructive invasion of the stroma and exhibits dense, confluent proliferation of glands with minimal stroma or absence of intervening stroma. The area of invasion must measure more than 10 mm^2 in area, or more than 3 mm in each of 2 linear dimensions.

The infiltrative pattern is considered more biologically aggressive than the expansile type. In 80% of cases, benign and borderline areas coexist with frankly malignant tissue.

Differential Diagnosis. This includes metastatic MA, which may have originated in the large intestine, appendix, pancreas, biliary tract, stomach or cervix; mucinous borderline tumors; endometrioid carcinoma with mucinous differentiation; Sertoli-Leydig tumors with heterologous mucinous component. Features that suggest the diagnosis of a metastatic origin include bilaterality, multinodular growth, superficial and extra ovarian dissemination, vascular invasions and central dirty necrosis and garland-like images.

Cytology. Cytological specimens show 2–3D irregular, dense cell clusters, sometimes with a papillary configuration, loosely cohesive sheets with slight loss of polarity and individual cells. Cells and nuclei vary in size and shape, and nuclear atypia tends to be moderate to high. Nuclei may be hyperchromatic, with coarsely granular chromatin and prominent nucleoli or macronucleoli. Uniform, regularly dispersed granular chromatin can also be seen. The background is mucinous, with hemorrhagic and necrotic tumor diathesis. The benign component is represented by monolayered sheets with a honeycomb pattern and a lack of nuclear atypia. Cellular cohesive 2–3D sheets, with low-to-moderate nuclear atypia and slight loss of polarity and isolated palisaded strips with nuclear stratification and hyperchromasia represent borderline areas that show sparse mitosis.

8.2.1.5. Mucinous Borderline Tumor

Mucinous bordeline tumor (MBT) is less frequent than SBT. Eighty per cent of the mucinous tumors are benign, while MBT are more frequent than invasive mucinous carcinomas. Two subtypes have been described: the intestinal type MBT and the endocervical-like type (EMBT) that is less common than the former. Extensive sampling of these tumors is very important, due to their histological heterogeneity. The known limitations of sampling in intraoperative procedures determine that the diagnosis to rule out invasion should be deferred to definitive paraffin sections.

Intestinal Type MBT. The gross examination shows large cystic tumors, averaging 20 cm in diameter, usually multilocular, with polypoid or papillary excrescences lining the internal surface either partially or totally. Microscopically cysts, glands and papillae are lined by cylindrical mucinous cells containing goblet cells. Two or three layers of epithelial stratification is the limit for the diagnosis of intestinal-type MBT. Nuclear atypia is low to moderate, with either very few or numerous mitoses. Stromal invasion is absent. The intraepithelial carcinoma areas have epithelial stratification of 4 or more layers, intraglandular or intraluminal proliferation of filiform branching papillae without stromal cores. There are also areas of complex glandular or cribriform pattern and moderate to high nuclear atypia These intraepithelial carcinoma areas have an upper limit of 10 square mm in size. MBT with intraepithelial carcinoma are considered clinically benign.

The favorable prognosis of intestinal type MBT is not altered by the presence of foci of stromal microinvasion showing confluent glands, aggregates of cribriform glands, small nests of cells occupying an area of 10 square mm in size or less than 3 mm in linear extent.

Endocervical-Like MBT. Endocervical-like MBT account for 10–15% of MBT. The average age is 40 years. Association with endometriosis has been reported, and dissemination to the peritoneum and lymph nodes may already be present by the time of the diagnosis.

Macroscopy. Forty percent of cases are reported as bilateral. Eighty percent are unilocular cysts showing intracystic papillae.

Microscopy. Microscopy reveals the presence of a complex papillary pattern similar to SBT. A careful search of mucinous columnar cells is necessary for diagnosis, as stratification and cellular budding may also be misleading. Cells with eosinophilic cytoplasm are seen in the tips of the papillae with tufting images. Neutrophils are present in the stroma and epithelium. Microinvasion and intraepithelial carcinoma is also described in this subtype.

Cytology. Cytological specimens of endocervical-like MBT show low to moderate cellularity with 2–3D dense cell groups, slightly loosely cohesive cell clusters, with some peripheral dissociation of cells and single cells. Palisaded strips with nuclear stratification and honeycomb sheets can be seen. Moderate nuclear atypia is usual but sometimes high nuclear atypia is present. Nuclei show granular, regularly distributed or coarse chromatin with hyperchromasia and single, fine, distinct nucleoli. Mitosis are rare. Nuclear and N/C ratio variability may be evident. A mucinous background is seen. In endocervical-like MBT, prominence of cells with abundant vacuolated cytoplasm, some of which have signet-ring-like configuration and neutrophils admixed with the epithelial elements and in the background is frequently found. The benign component is represented by few clusters and monolayered sheets of epithelial cells with a honeycomb pattern and palisaded strips with basally oriented nuclei and absence of nuclear atypia. Histiocytes may also be observed (fig. 8.10–8.12).

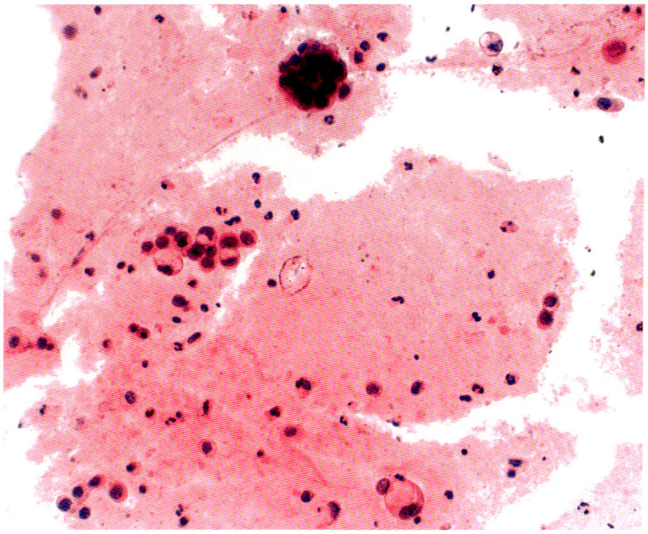

Fig. 8.10. Mucinous borderline tumor, endocervical-like. Two- and three-dimensional dense cellular groups. Low to moderate nuclear atypia. Vacuolated cytoplasm. Mucinous background. HE, 20×.

8.2.1.6. Endometrioid Tumors

These ovarian tumors resemble those of the endometrium. Recent molecular studies suggest that most endometrial carcinomas arise from the malignant transformation of endometriosis, and not from the ovarian surface epithelium. They represent from 2 to 5% of all ovarian tumors.

Endometrioid tumors have benign, borderline and malignant subtypes. Benign endometrioid tumors are very rare (less than 1% of all benign tumors of the ovary), presenting as adenofibromas, and their epithelial lining is similar to proliferative or inactive endometrium. Borderline subtypes represent 2–3% of ovarian borderline tumors, and present as adenofibromas or cystadenofibromas. A histologically

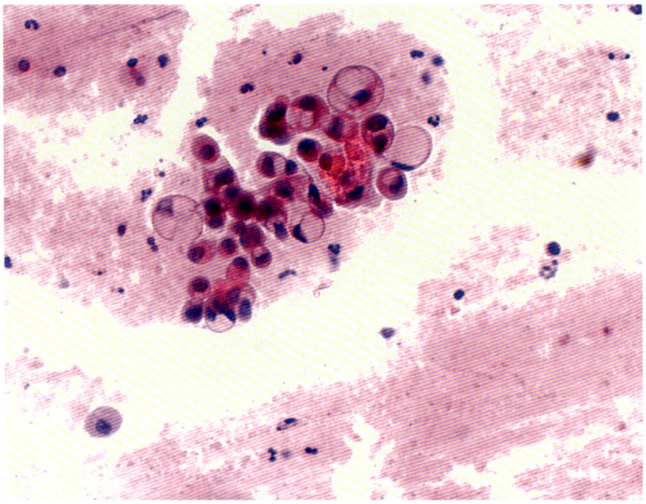

Fig. 8.11. Mucinous borderline tumor, endocervical-like. Cellular aggregates with loss of polarity and cohesiveness. Peripheral dispersion of nuclei and cells. Moderate nuclear atypia, vacuolated cytoplasm. Mucinous, granular background. HE, 20×.

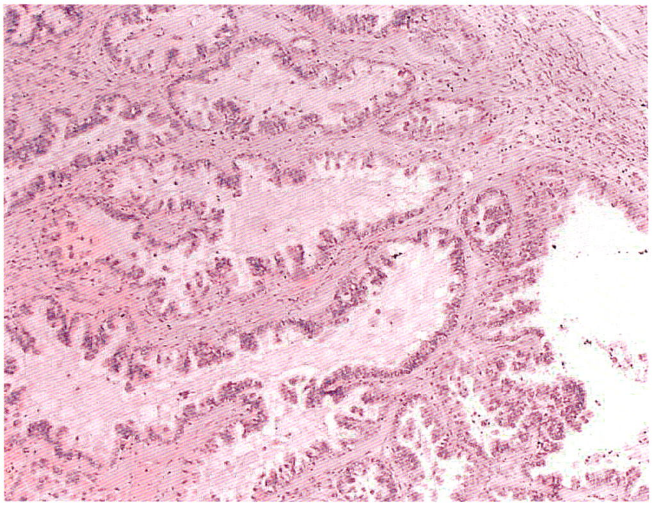

Fig. 8.12. Mucinous borderline tumor, endocervical-like. Complex papillary pattern. Cellular budding. Neutrophils in the stroma and epithelium. Variable nuclear atypia. HE, 4×.

complex or atypical hyperplasia with intraepithelial carcinoma of the epithelial endometrial component can be observed. The same parameters as in the endometrium are used to diagnose these lesions. The prognosis is favorable.

Endometrioid Carcinoma. Endometrioid carcinoma represents 80% of endometrioid tumors and 10–20% of ovarian carcinomas. It ranks second in frequency in the category of epithelial carcinomas. In 28% of the cases it is bilateral. Histologically endometrioid carcinoma are predominantly well to moderately differentiated carcinomas and they may show associated epithelial changes like secretory and squamous differentiation. Onset is during the 5th or 6th decades of life, although when associated with ovarian endometriosis the average age is 5–10 years younger, and they are usually low grade and diagnosed at an early stage. In 15–20% of cases endometrioid carcinoma is associated with carcinoma of the endometrium.

Favorable prognosis is related to 70% of the cases diagnosed at stage I.

Macroscopy. Gross appearance is predominantly cystic, with papillary and friable nodular masses protruding into the cystic lumen. Hemorrhagic fluid is commonly found. Thick-walled cysts point to endometrioid carcinoma's origin in an endometriotic cyst. Some tumors are solid, presenting with hemorrhage and necrosis.

Microscopy. Well-differentiated endometrioid carcinoma show glandular, papillary, cribriform and villoglandular patterns. Round, oval or tubular glands are lined by stratified columnar epithelium. Endometrioid cells have small dark nuclei with scanty and/or vacuolated cytoplasm. A regular number of mitosis are found, showing up to 5 mitoses per 10 high-power fields. Squamous differentiation occurs in 30–50% of the cases. Morules with cytologically benign squamous elements may also be present. When squamous malignant elements are intermingled with the glandular component, the tumors are designated as EdC with squamous differentiation. The presence of mucin and secretory, ciliated, microglandular patterns, as well as sex-cord like tubular areas is commonly reported. Other epithelial types, such as clear cell adenocarcinoma and serous carcinoma are seen in up to 30% of the tumors.

Poorly differentiated carcinomas have a solid pattern with focal glandular areas presenting with moderate to high nuclear atypia. Mitosis can be observed in numerous cells.

Cytology. Cytological specimens show 2–3D spherical aggregates and large, crowded cellular sheets with slight loss of cohesiveness and polarity. Peripheral dissociation of cells in the groups is typical. Scattered single cells are present. Cytology shows small- and medium-sized atypical cells, with round-to-oval and slightly enlarged hyperchromatic nuclei, presenting with finely granular and evenly distributed chromatin and small distinct nucleoli. The cytoplasm is scanty, sometimes vacuolated, and its borders are ill-defined, resulting in high N/C ratios. Mitosis are rare. A few oval and spindle-shaped stromal cells with an indistinct or scant cytoplasm and small oval nuclei can be found in loose monolayered sheets.

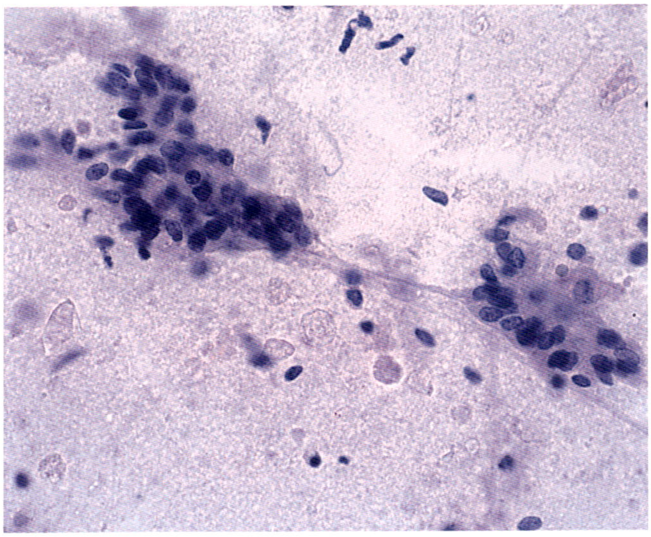

Fig. 8.13. Endometrioid carcinoma. Three-dimensional crowded cellular groups and individual cells. Loss of polarity and cohesiveness. Moderate nuclear atypia, granular chromatin, small nucleoli and scanty cytoplasm. HE, 20×.

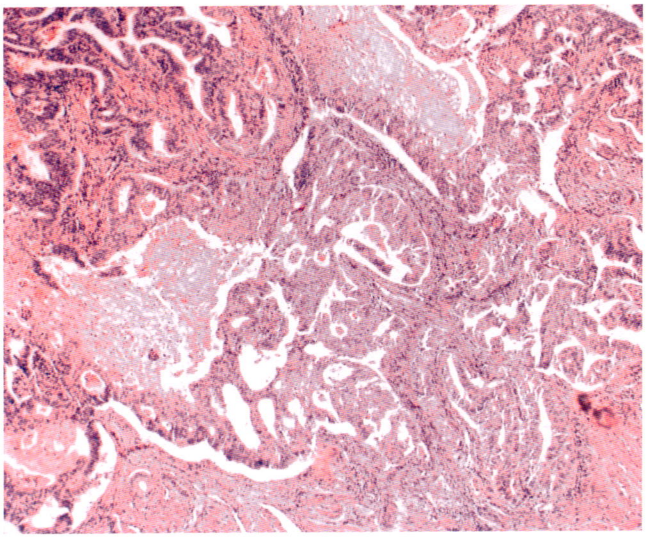

Fig. 8.15. Endometrioid carcinoma with squeamous differentiation. HE, 4×.

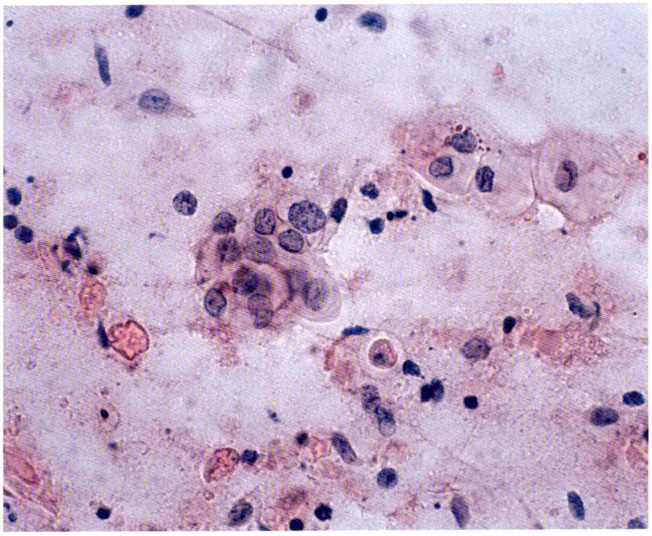

Fig. 8.14. Endometrioid carcinoma with squamous differentiation. Sheet-like apithelial clusters with abundant dense eosinophilic cytoplasm and distinct cellular borders. Moderate nuclear atypia. HE, 40×.

In poorly differentiated carcinomas smears show high cellularity. Cell aggregates are loosely cohesive with loss of polarity and there are numerous single cells. The enlarged nuclei show irregular sizes and shapes, exhibiting hyperchromatic nuclei with granular irregular chromatin and distinct fine nucleoli. The tumor background tends to be hemorrhagic, with or without necrosis.

In endometrioid carcinomas with squamous differentiation, squamous cells show dense eosinophilic or at times clear cytoplasm with well-defined borders. Nuclei have coarse, granular and irregular chromatin (fig. 8.13 –8.15).

8.2.1.7. Clear Cell Carcinoma

Clear cell tumors are classified as benign, borderline and malignant subtypes. Benign clear cell tumors are very rare, presenting as adenofibromas. Borderline subtypes represent less than 1% of the borderline ovarian tumors and clear cell carcinomas account for 6% of the ovarian epithelial cancers.

They occur in the 5th to 7th decades of life, and 50% are diagnosed in stage 1. They are strongly associated with endometriosis in 40–60% of cases, i.e. more frequently than endometrioid carcinoma. In some areas, cystic endometriosis may coexist with clear cell carcinomas. Association of simultaneous endometrioid carcinoma and clear cell carcinomas of the uterus and ovary occurs in 20–25% of the cases.

Macroscopy. Gross examination shows large cystic tumors, measuring 15–20 cm in diameter. Focal or diffuse polypoid excrescences are frequently present in the cyst's inner surface, with areas of necrosis and hemorrhage. The content is commonly a hemorrhagic or clear fluid. Ten percent of these tumors are bilateral.

Microscopy. The coexistence of solid, tubulocystic and tubulo-papillary patterns is frequent. Uniform

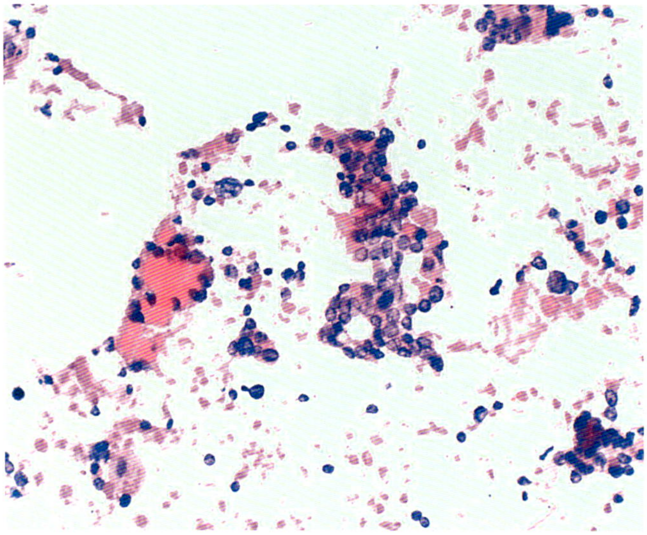

Fig. 8.16. Clear cell carcinoma. High cellularity. Loosely cohesive cell clusters. Uniform, small, round, papillary groups. Individual cells. Eosinophilic secretion. HE, 20×.

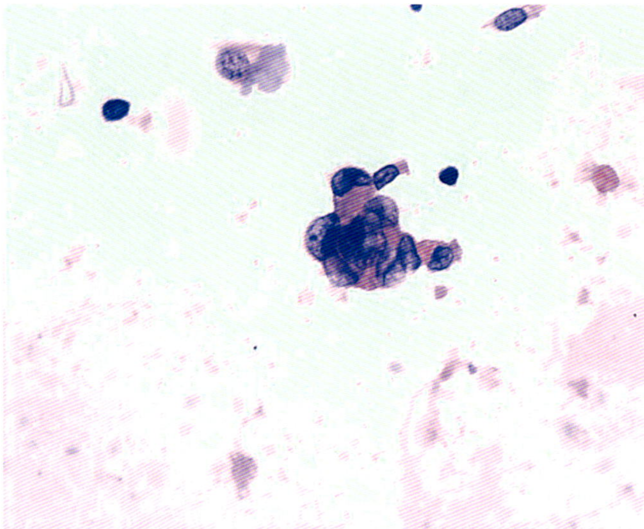

Fig. 8.17. Clear cell carcinoma. Three-dimensional papillary group. Nuclear protusion in hobnail cells. High nuclear atypia, hyperchromasia. Vacuolated cytoplasm. HE, 40×.

homogeneous-sized, small and round papillae with hyalinized stromal cores are typically observed. It is also common to find hyalinized homogenous eosinophilic material expanding the cores of the papillae or occupying the stroma. Solid epithelial aggregates are divided by delicate fibrovascular septa. Cells have an abundant and clear glycogenic cytoplasm, and distinct cell borders. Some cells have intracytoplasmatic hyaline eosinophilic globules, a feature that helps in the diagnosis.

Round, vesicular and eccentric nuclei with moderate-to-high nuclear atypia and prominent nucleoli are found. Mitosis are rare, usually showing fewer than 2 per 10 high-power fields. The fibrous stroma shows hyalinization and scanty microcalcifications. Necrosis, hemorrhage and lymphoid infiltrates may be present as well. Hobnail cells typically show apical protrusion of their nuclei. Oxyphilic cells with abundant eosinophilic cytoplasm and signet-ring cells can also be found.

Differential Diagnosis. This includes disgerminoma, yolk-sac tumor, juvenile granulosa cell tumor, Krukenberg tumor, metastatic renal cell carcinoma, Arias-Stella reaction, steroid cell tumor, endometrial adenocarcinoma with secretory changes or squamous differentiation with cytoplasmic glycogen.

Cytology. Cytological specimens show monolayers of loosely cohesive sheets or 3-dimensional groups and numerous usually even-sized, small papillary aggregates with hyaline stromal cores, as those seen in histology. Single cells are found, and the cytoplasm of epithelial cells may be abundant and clear or finely granular and ill defined. High nuclear atypia with granular chromatin, prominent nucleoli and scarce macronucleoli may be observed. The nuclear/cytoplasmic ratio is relatively low. Hobnail cells show apical protrusion of nuclei. Some cells show clear vesicular nuclei with marginal clumping of chromatin and irregular nuclear membranes. Mitosis are rare. Tumor diathesis in which hyalinized eosinophilic homogenous material is seen lying free in the background, constitutes a characteristic feature (fig. 8.16–8.18).

8.2.1.8. Benign Brenner Tumor

Benign Brenner tumors represent less than 5% of the benign epithelial-stromal tumors. Usually asymptomatic, they are found incidentally in ovaries removed for some other reason. Patient age ranges from 30 to 60 years.

Macroscopy. Half of them are grossly visible, with sizes ranging between 2 and 10 cm. Less than 10% are bilateral. Gross features are brownish, nodular, sharply circumscribed, capsule-free fibrous masses. Small cysts and focal calcification are common. Cystic mucinous differentiation can appear mixed to the benign tumor mass.

Microscopy. Round-to-oval epithelial nests or trabeculae of mature transitional cells can be seen within a fibromatous stroma. Epithelial cells show a round-to-polygonal configuration with eosinophilic or clear cytoplasm and distinct cell membranes. Nuclei are oval and bland with

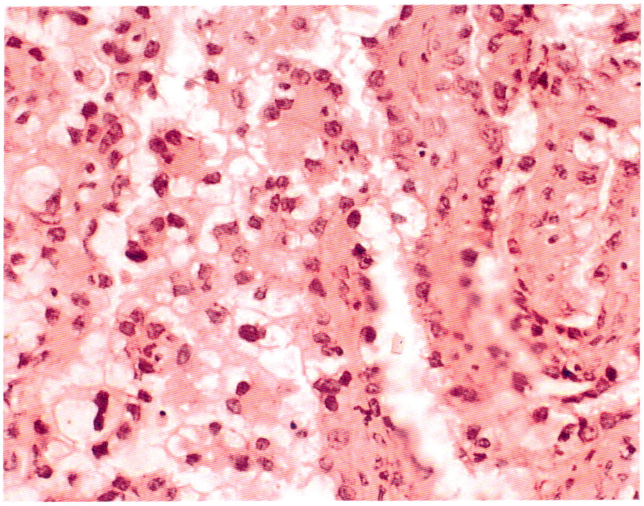

Fig. 8.18. Clear cell carcinoma. Solid, papillary pattern. Clear cells with high nuclear atypia, prominent nucleoli and vacuolated cytoplasm. HE, 20×.

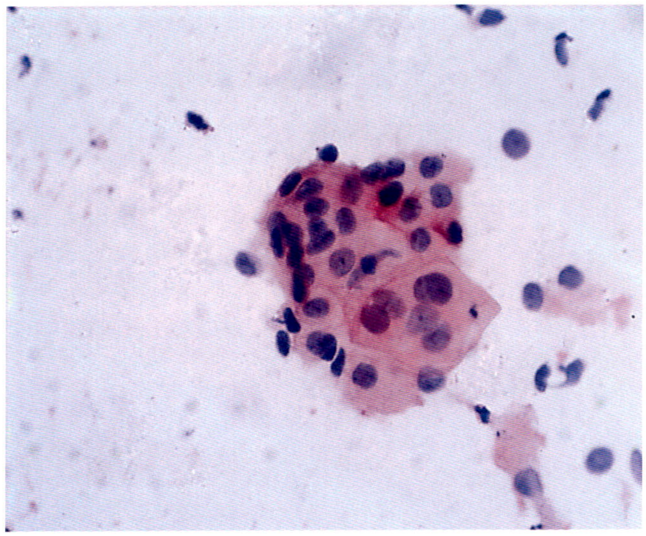

Fig. 8.20. Benign Brenner tumor. Aggregate of epithelial cells, with ovoid, bland nuclei, longitudinal grooves and fine nucleoli. Ample eosinophilic cytoplasm with distinct cell membranes. HE, 40×.

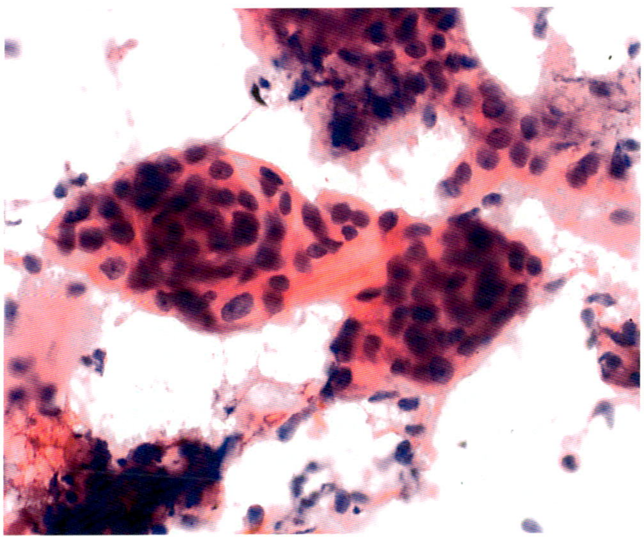

Fig. 8.19. Benign Brenner tumor. Three-dimensional dense clusters of epithelial transitional cells. Ovoid to round, bland nuclei with fine chromatin and distinct nucleoli. HE, 40×.

fine, evenly dispersed chromatin, obvious nucleoli and a frequent longitudinal grooving that gives them a coffee-bean appearance. Mitoses are rare. Epithelial nests may have a central cavity containing densely eosinophilic, mucin-positive material and lined with mucinous, ciliated serous or indifferent epithelium. Squamous differentiation may be found in the nests. Large cysts may be lined with transitional or mucinous epithelium. The stroma may be typical of an ovarian fibroma/thecoma, and it may contain luteinized cells. Hyalinization and dystrophic calcification may be present.

Cytology. Cytological specimens show a clean background with numerous spindle/fibrous non-atypical cells. Three-dimensional epithelial cell nests are identified. Epithelial cells have a dense and abundant eosinophilic cytoplasm with well-defined cell borders. Nuclei are bland, ovoid or round in shape and the longitudinal groove that gives them a coffee-bean like appearance seen in the histology may be observed. Fine regular chromatin and small distinct nucleoli are also typical findings. An intraluminal eosinophilic mucus substance is seen within cavitated cell nests or lying free in the background (fig. 8.19–8.21).

8.2.2. Metastatic Tumors

Between 6 and 20% of ovarian malignant tumors are metastatic. Patients with metastasis to the ovary are younger than women with primary ovarian tumors. Primary tumors arising from the stomach, breast, intestine, appendix, genital tract, and melanoma, among others, can metastasize the ovaries. Prognosis is poor, with a 12% overall 5-year survival rate.

Macroscopy. Typical gross features of metastatic tumors are bilaterality and multinodularity of solid masses.

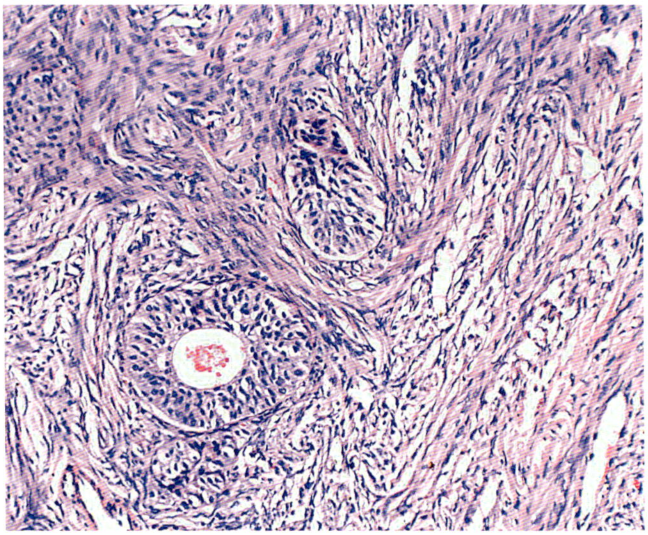

Fig. 8.21. Benign Brenner tumor. Nests of transitional cells and fibromatous stroma. Epithelial nests with central cavities and dense eosinophilic material. HE, 10×.

Bilaterality is seen in over 50% of the cases. Unilateral tumors smaller than 10 cm are usually metastatic [21]. Cystic or partially cystic tumors may occur, and necrosis and hemorrhage are frequent findings. The outer surface may be smooth or it may show the presence of nodular masses.

Microscopy. The microscopic appearance depends on the histology of the primary tumors. The growth pattern is characteristically multinodular, with tumor cells, small glands and tubules and single cells infiltrating a desmoplastic stroma that may present with variable amounts of dense, fibrous areas. Foci of stromal luteinization may also be seen, and the invasion of blood and lymphatic vessels in the periphery of the tumor is common. The gross or microscopic involvement of the ovarian surface is a frequent finding, while the sparing of follicular structures is a useful diagnostic clue. Small tumors are confined to the medulla.

8.2.2.1. Metastasis from Colon and Rectum

Macroscopy. The gross examination shows large, lobulated and multinodular, bilateral tumors. The solid masses may host cystic spaces with necrotic debris and mucinous fluid. Surface adhesions may be present.

Microscopy. The histological glandular and cribriform pattern mimics a primary endometrial adenocarcinoma. Individual glands with segmental necrosis of the epithelial lining and necrosis in tumor nodules that leave a peripheral rim of viable epithelium are responsible for the garland-like images observed, which contain necrotic debris, or 'dirty necrosis'. The high nuclear atypia is a helpful clue to differentiate it from a primary ovarian adenocarcinoma. Mucin secretion is seen in the apical cytoplasm and gland lumens. The amount of stroma is variable and there may be luteinized cells present.

Differential Diagnosis. Mucinous primary tumors, endometrioid, clear cell carcinomas.

Cytology. Cytological specimens show high cellularity, abundant mucin and a necrotic, hemorrhagic tumor background, as well as single cells and numerous cell clusters showing loss of cohesion and polarity. There is usually a high nuclear atypia, with obvious variations in size and shape, irregular nuclear membranes and prominent nucleoli and macro-nucleoli. The cytoplasm is vacuolated or granular, with well-defined borders.

8.2.2.2. Krukenberg Tumors

Krukenberg tumors account for 3–8% of all carcinomas metastasizing the ovaries. Seventy-six percent originate in the stomach, 11% in the intestines, 3% in the biliary system, 3% in the appendix and 3% in miscellaneous sites (pancreas, uterine cervix, urinary bladder and renal pelvis). The typical pattern of these tumors consists of the presence of a component of epithelial signet-ring mucin cells infiltrating a fibrous stroma. There must be no evidence of any other primary neoplasms with signet ring cells.

Macroscopy. Eighty percent of these tumors are bilateral, and they present with a bosselated, smooth, external surface. The cut surface shows a solid nodular, white-to-yellow tan mass with red-purple focal areas. The consistency of the tumors is soft, spongy and gelatinous, due to edema and the mucinous content. Cystic degeneration may occur. Average size is up to 10 cm.

Microscopy. Epithelial cells with dense and eosinophilic cytoplasm and signet-ring cells with pale, vacuolated cytoplasm, and hyperchromatic, eccentric nuclei are observed. The pattern of growth is in nodular nests, trabeculae or single cells infiltrating a fibrous stroma with variable cellularity. Edema and pools of mucin may be present in the stroma. The number of signet-ring epithelial cells also varies, being in some cases very numerous. When they are scarce and inconspicuous, and located in the midst of a densely cellular fibrous stroma, the diagnosis is quite challenging. Small- to medium-sized glands are found and, less frequently, a tubular pattern is seen. Blood vessel and lymphatic invasion is common, and mitotic activity is low.

Differential Diagnosis. Clear cell carcinoma, mucinous carcinoids, Sertoli-Leydig tumors and sclerosing stromal tumors.

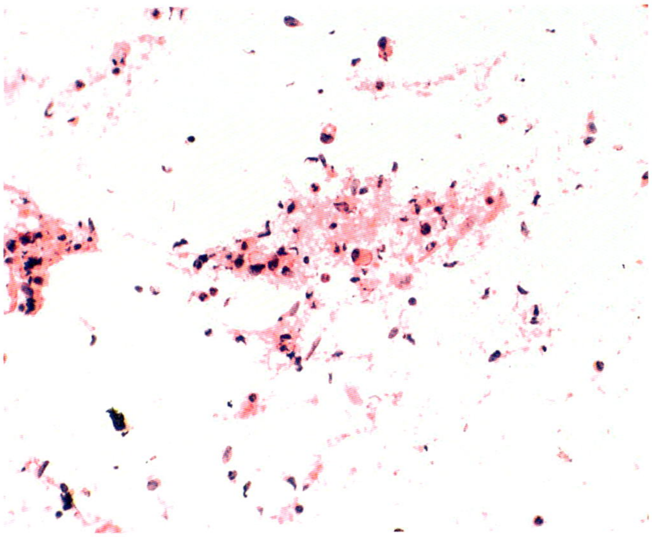

Fig. 8.22. Krukenberg tumor. Scarce signet-ring cells with eccentric, hyperchromatic nuclei, ample vacuolated cytoplasm and high nuclear atypia. Individual spindle stromal cells. Tumoral background. HE, 20×.

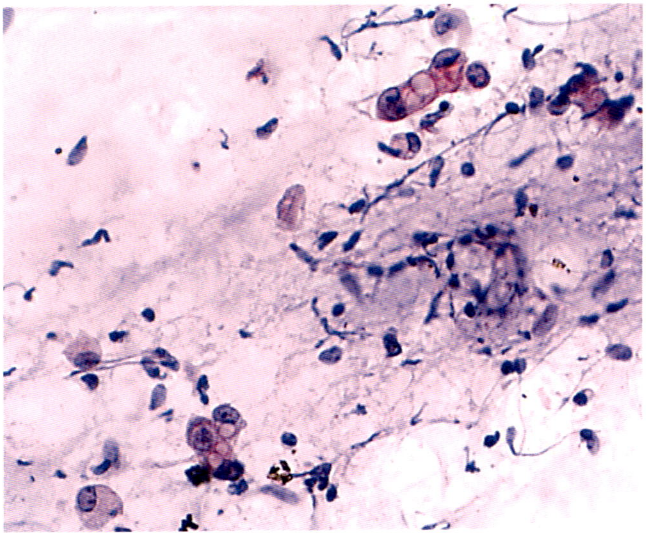

Fig. 8.23. Krukenberg tumor. Numerous signet-ring cells with high N/C ratios, prominent nucleoli. Spindle stromal cells. Tumoral background. HE, 20×.

Cytology. Specimens are difficult to evaluate when there is fibrotic stroma overgrowth with scarce epithelial cells. In these cases, there may be a tumor background with necrosis and hemorrhage and numerous spindle-shaped, fibroblastic-like cells and very scarce, scattered signet-ring and malignant epithelial cells. The fibrous stromal cells have ovoid bland, non-atypical nuclei, with scant, elongated cytoplasm. The epithelial signet-ring cells have eccentric hyperchromatic nuclei, prominent nucleoli and pale vacuolated cytoplasm, and high nuclear atypia.

In Krukenberg tumors with high cellularity smears, the numerous typical signet-ring cells with pale vacuolated cytoplasm are easy to find (fig. 8.22, 8.23).

8.2.3. Non-Neoplastic Cysts

8.2.3.1. Endometriotic Cysts

Macroscopy. Endometriotic cysts with a hemorrhagic content must be distinguished from other functional hemorrhagic cysts, such as the corpus luteum cyst, follicular cysts and cystic benign or malignant epithelial tumors. Among the latter, endometrioid, clear cell, serous and mucinous malignant tumors may be cystic and hemorrhagic, while borderline tumors are less frequently hemorrhagic. Granulosa cell tumor and Sertoli-Leydig tumors may also occur in a cystic and hemorrhagic variant. The thick, fibrous, red-brown colored wall suggests an endometriotic origin.

Microscopy. The positive diagnosis of an ovarian endometriotic cyst requires the identification of endometrial epithelium on the wall lining or in the glandular component and/or the presence of endometrial stroma. The endometrial epithelium consists of tall, columnar cells with pseudo stratified elongated, ovoid nuclei, and scanty cytoplasm. Glands are usually inactive and the stroma shows small spindle cells with inconspicuous cytoplasm and the presence of focal or diffuse hemosiderin-laden macrophages. The fibrous hemorrhagic cystic walls are frequently denuded of their internal epithelial lining. Multiple frozen or paraffin sections are generally needed for a correct diagnosis. Deferral of intraoperative consultation may be reasonable.

Cytology. Cytological specimens show a hemorrhagic background. Numerous hemosiderin-laden macrophages are found with abundant, foamy, lightly eosinophilic granular cytoplasm and round-to-ovoid bland nuclei, with fine prominent nucleoli. Endometrial cells are observed in scattered 2D, cohesive groups or monolayered sheets of small cells with scanty cytoplasm are found. Nuclei are uniform, dark-stained and round-to-oval with inconspicuous nucleoli. Polarity is preserved and there is no evidence of mitosis. Some endometrial cells may present degenerative-type nuclear atypia, not to be confused with malignant cells. Scarce spindle stromal cells in loose monolayered sheets with indistinct or scant cytoplasm and small oval nuclei can also be found (fig. 8.24, 8.25).

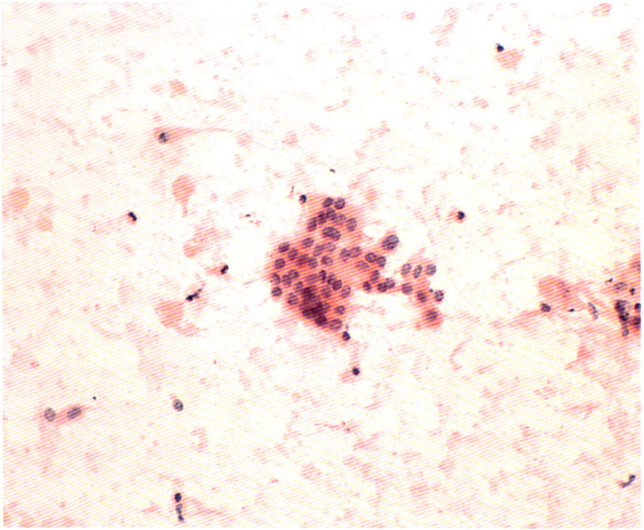

Fig. 8.24. Endometriotic cyst. Two-dimensional cohesive cellular group with small, uniform cells. Scanty cytoplasm, dark nuclei. HE, 20×.

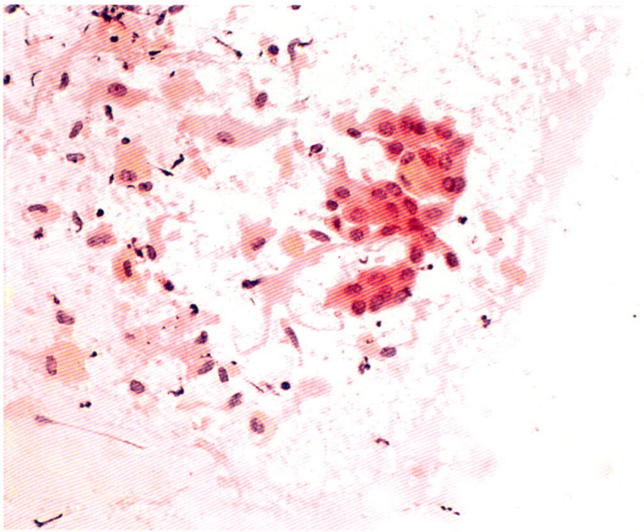

Fig. 8.25. Endometriotic cyst. Numerous hemosiderin-laden macrophages. Epithelial cells with abundant eosinophilic cytoplasm with reactive or smudged nuclei. HE, 20×.

8.2.3.2. Corpus Luteum Cyst

A cystic hemorrhagic corpus luteum may sometimes reach 10 cm or more in diameter, and it should be differentiated from the previously described neoplastic and non-neoplastic cystic hemorrhagic tumors. The external surface is usually smooth and free from any adhesions. The cut surface of the thin wall shows a typical yellow rim. Histology shows a convoluted luteinized inner lining consisting of granulosa and theca cells and the typical peripheral vascular zone. Luteinized cells have ample, finely granular cytoplasms and eccentric bland nuclei, round to oval, with small fine nucleoli. Absence of mitosis.

Cytology. Cytological specimens show individual or small groups of luteinized cells and red blood cells, hemosiderin-laden macrophages and scattered spindle, fibroblastic cells. Luteinized cells have ample finely granular or small vacuolated cyanophilic cytoplasm and nuclei are bland, with delicate, regular fine membranes and small but obvious nucleoli (fig. 8.26).

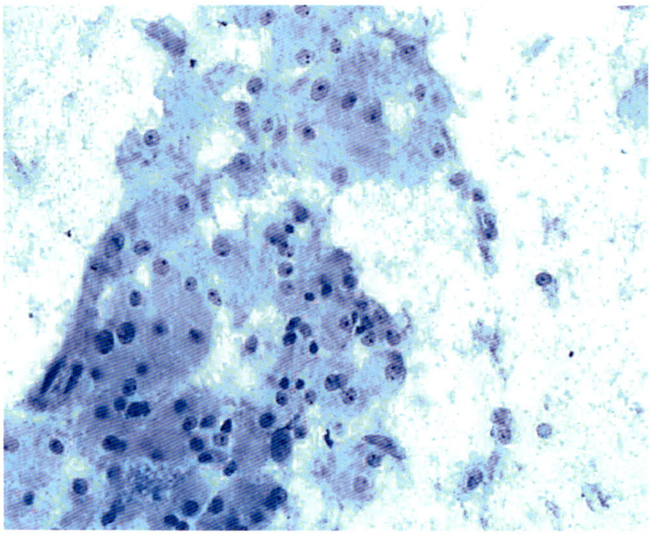

Fig. 8.26. Corpus luteum cyst. Luteinized cells with ample cytoplasm. Bland, oval and round nuclei, small nucleoli. HE, 10×.

8.2.4. Sex Cord-Stromal Tumors

8.2.4.1. Granulosa-Stromal Cell Tumor

Granulosa-stromal cell tumors are found in all ages and more frequently in young patients. They may be associated with hormonal symptoms, especially estrogen activity. The juvenile granulosa tumor occurs after puberty associated with isosexual precocity.

Macroscopy. Adult granulosa cell tumor is typically unilateral (95%). This tumor varies in size, with an average of approximately 12 cm, it is encapsulated and tends to be soft and fleshy. The outer surface is smooth and lobulated. The cut section shows a solid surface and cystic areas with serous

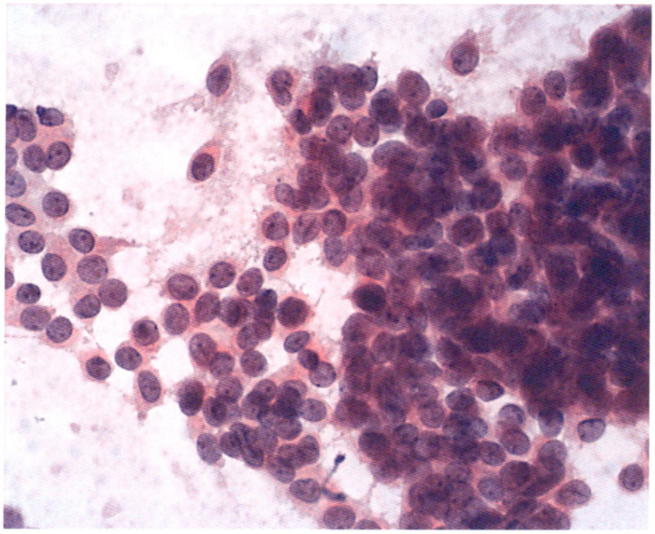

Fig. 8.27. Granulosa cell tumor, adult type. Monolayared and two-dimensional dense cell clusters. Individual cells. Uniform small round to ovoid nuclei. Nuclear grooves. Prominent nucleoli. Scant cytoplasm. HE, 20×.

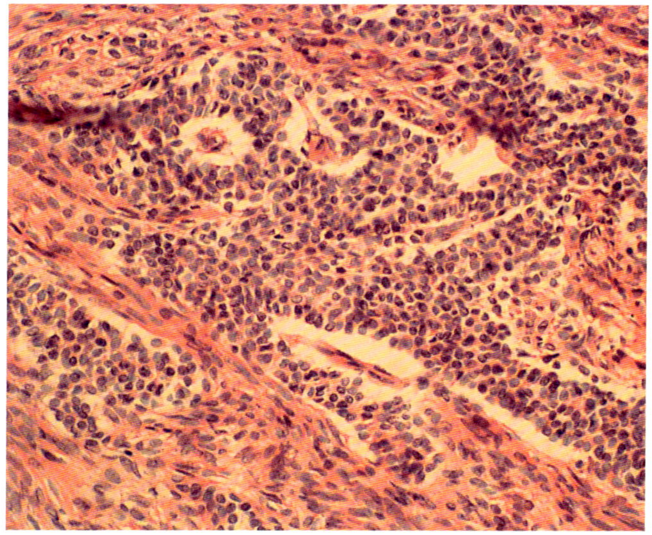

Fig. 8.28. Granulosa cell tumor, adult type. Trabecular and microfollicular pattern. Call-Exner bodies containing eosinophilic material. Granulosa cells with ovoid, grooved nuclei in a fibromatous stroma. HE, 20×.

or hemorrhagic contents. The white, yellow or brownish color is a typical characteristic of steroid-secreting tumors, reflecting lipid-rich contents.

Bulky tumors usually show hemorrhage, cystic cavities filled with hemorrhagic contents and, less frequently, necrosis.

Microscopy. The proliferation of granulosa cells is admixed with a stromal fibroadenomatous component where theca or luthenized cells may be found. The adult granulosa cell tumor variant is the most frequent and shows a range of histological patterns, including solid, trabecular, insular, follicular, gyriform and diffuse (sarcomatoid). The follicular pattern sometime shows rosette-like structures known as Call-Exner bodies, which resemble primitive follicles.

The granulosa cells present round and ovoid nuclei with longitudinal grooves and scant cytoplasm. The lutheinized cells have an abundant eosinophilic or vacuolated cytoplasm with rounded nuclei without grooves. The presence of bizarre nuclei has no adverse effects on prognosis.

The juvenile variant of the granulosa cell tumor shows a solid growth pattern with follicle formation with irregular sizes and shapes. Cells have round, hyperchromatic nuclei, usually without longitudinal grooves. Mild to marked atypia and abundant eosinophilic or vacuolated cytoplasm (luthenized) is found.

Differential Diagnosis. Undifferentiated carcinoma, endometrioid adenocarcinoma, carcinoid and luteinized thecoma.

Cytology. Cytological specimens of adult granulosa cell tumor show a clean background with high cellularity. Dense, mono-layered, 2-dimensional cell clusters and single cells, as well as rosette-like clusters that correspond to Call-Exner bodies are found. The cells have uniform, round to ovoid, angulated nuclei with fine, regular chromatin, small prominent nucleoli and scanty cytoplasm. The N/C ratio is high and longitudinal nuclear grooves are typically observed. Nuclei are bland or hyperchromatic (fig. 8.27, 8.28).

8.2.4.2. Typical and Luteinized Thecoma

Typical thecoma is one third as common as granulosa cell tumor. Most of them (84%) are observed in menopausal patients, with a mean age of 59 years. Thecomas are rare before puberty and only 10% occur in women under 30 years of age. The rare lutheinized thecoma variant, associated with sclerosing peritonitis typically occurs in older women.

Macroscopy. The tumor diameter is usually 5–10 cm. The cut surface is yellowish, solid and firm and it has clear-cut limits, occasionally presenting with cysts, hemorrhage and necrosis.

Microscopy. It is benign stromal tumor with lipid-containing cells similar to the inner theca cells, with a variable fibroblast component.

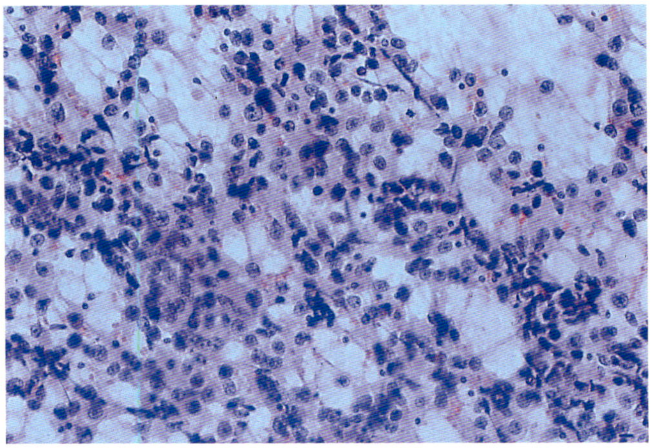

Fig. 8.29. Dysgerminoma. High cellularity. Large, uniform, individual tumor cells. Round, vesicular nuclei with granular, coarse chromatin and prominent nucleoli. Numerous small lymphocytes. Tumoral background. HE, 10×.

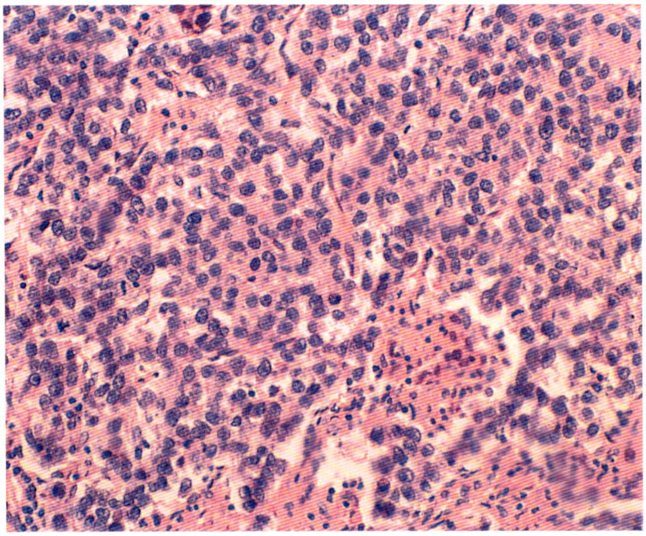

Fig. 8.30. Dysgerminoma. Large uniform tumoral cells. High nuclear atypia, prominent nucleoli, mitosis. Granular cytoplasm, indistinct cell borders. Connective tissue septa, lymphocytes. HE, 20×.

Its growth pattern shows well-defined solid nodules, separated by connective tissue bands. The theca cells are round or elongated, with soft, uniform, ovoid or spindle-shaped central nuclei, with no grooves, and abundant eosinophilic or vacuolated cytoplasm. Reticuline fibers surround the cells individually. The fibromatous component commonly contains hyaline plaques and it may also present focal calcifications. Rarely, large or bizarre nuclei are found, but they do not have prognostic significance.

Cytology. Cytological specimens show a clean background where elongated, spindle-shaped cells resembling fibroblasts are seen. They have small, ovoid, elongated or round, bland nuclei, with no longitudinal grooves. Chromatin is delicate, fine and regularly distributed, and nucleoli are inconspicuous.

8.2.5. Germ Cell Tumors

8.2.5.1. Dysgerminoma

Dysgerminoma. This is the most frequent primitive malignant germ cell tumor. It accounts for 1% of all the ovarian cancers, and 5–10% of all ovarian cancers presenting in the first 20 years of life. Eighty percent are observed between 20 and 30 years of age.

Macroscopy. Most of these tumors are round and solid, with a smooth white-to-grayish outer surface. They vary in size and have an average diameter up to 15 cm and may weigh over 5 kg. Fifteen percent are bilateral. The cut surface is solid and pinkish grey. There is evidence of necrosis and hemorrhage and sometimes cysts are found, especially in the largest ones.

Microscopy. They present a growth pattern with cords, and nests of tumor cells that vary in size, separated by connective tissue septa with lymphocytes, sometimes plasma cells, histiocytes and eosinophiles. The tumor cells are large, polygonal and uniformly sized, with round nuclei, angulated at times, prominent nucleoli and a granular cytoplasm. Isolated syncitiotrophoblast cells can also be observed.

Cytology. Cytological specimens show high cellularity with large, uniform, isolated tumor cells and numerous small benign lymphocytes. Plasma cells and hystiocytes may also be found. Tumor cells have round, vesicular nuclei, presenting with glanular, coarse, irregularly distributed chromatin and prominent single or multiple nucleoli and moderate amounts of pale, granular cytoplasm. A tumoral background with hemorrhage and necrosis is found (fig. 8.29, 8.30).

8.3. Performance of Intraoperative Cytology

Although pathologists seem to have a higher level of confidence in frozen sections in the intraoperative consultation, several authors [9–11, 14, 15, 20, 23, 25] have recently reported their performance using cytology in routine practice (table 8.1). The number of ovarian cases reported in the 8 series reviewed is limited, ranging from 10–617 cases. Some of the reports calculate diagnostic accuracy using

Table 8.1. Comparison between intraoperative cytology and frozen section plus cytology for definitive paffin diagnosis

Study	Year	Cases, n	Diagnostic accuracy, %			
			IOC		FS + IOC	
Souka et al. [25]	1990	50[1]	B + M	84.0		90.0
Ittee [10]	1993	10/80[2]	B + M	92.5	B + M	78.8
			B	90.6		
			M	93.7		
Scucchi et al. [20]	1997	2,250[2]	B + M	96.0	B + M	99.2
Shidham et al. [23]	2000	14/446[2]	B	96.0	B + M	93.7
			M	91.2		
Nagai et al. [15]	2001	354[1]	B	87.1		
			Bl.	30.0		
			M	89.5		
Khunamornpong and Siriaunkgul [11]	2003	131[1]	B.	95.0		
			Bl	47.0		
			M	98.0		
Ilvan et al. [9]	2005	617[1]			B + M	97
					B	99
					BL	97
					M	97
Alvarez Santín [2]	2009	337[1]	B + M	98.5	B + M	95.2
			B	100	B	96.0
					Bl.	80.0
			M	92.7	M	87.7

B = Benign; Bl. = borderline; FA = frozen section; IOC = intraoperative cytology; M = malignant.
[1] Ovary
[2] Various organs

only cytology specimens, while others report their results with the simultaneous use of cytology and frozen sections. Reports on the accuracy of intraoperative cytology in benign and/or malignant tumors range from 84–100%, with the exception of the borderline category which has a much lower performance. The high accuracy recorded underscore the role of intraoperative cytological diagnosis in ovarian lesions.

8.4. Advantages and Limitations

The objective of intraoperative consultation in cases of ovarian tumors is to determine the malignant, primary or metastatic nature of the tumor and its histologic type and stage as a guide to further surgical management. Evaluation of macroscopic features and frozen sections is the traditional practice. The known limitations of frozen-section diagnosis, due to technical, sampling and interpretation problems can be partially overcome by including intraoperative cytological diagnosis and performing cyto-histologic correlation in the intraoperative consultation.

Obtaining cytological specimens has the advantage of being a simple and rapid method. Due to its rapid processing, cytology slides are ready first for diagnosis. In the case of large ovarian tumors, cytology specimens make possible the sampling of various sites, increasing cellular representation of the lesion, helping to overcome the limitation resulting from the limited number of tissue samples that can be processed and examined by frozen section during the rapid intraoperative procedure.

Cytology specimens ensure excellent preservation of cytological details in which the architecture of cell aggregates and nuclear and cytoplasmic features are easily evaluated. Cytohistological correlations can be performed, adding information to achieve a more precise diagnostic definition.

Limitations relate to the impossibility of performing counting and measurement procedures for diagnosis and grading tumors to evaluate stromal invasion, depth of tumor infiltration and – with some exceptions – of status of margin resection. Frequently, these limitations are also shared by frozen sections.

Although pathologists consider frozen sections to be the gold standard for intraoperative diagnosis, cytology may be the only diagnostic tool available when frozen section diagnosis fails due to technical, sampling or interpretation problems.

8.5. Conclusions

The advantages that have been described highlight the improved performance in intraoperative diagnosis that can be obtained by the simultaneous use of cytology specimens and frozen sections. Cytological smears represent an important complementary diagnostic tool in this context. The pathologist using this technique must have experience and proficiency in cytopathology and in this interesting pathologic field to achieve the high level of performance required of intraoperative consultations.

References

1 Acs G: Intraoperative consultation in gynecologic pathology. Semin Diagn Pathol 2002;19:237–254.
2 Alvarez Santín C: Cytopathology of ovarian endometrial Related Lesions. Cytopathology 2009; Suppl 1:29.
3 Baker P, Oliva E: A Practical Approach to Intraoperative consultation in Gynecological Pathology. Int J Gynecol Pathol 2008;27:353–365.
4 Bell D: Mucinous Ovarian Tumors. IAP 2004 Annual Congress. www.uscap.org/site/iap2004.
5 Bibbo M, Wood MD, Fitzpatrick BT: Peritoneal washings and ovary; in Bibbo M, Wilbur DC (eds): Comprehensive Cytopathology, ed 3. Amsterdam, Elsevier, 2008, pp 294–299.
6 Geisinger KR, Stanley MW, Stephen SR, Silverman JF, Abati A: The pelvis and scrotal contents; in: Modern Cytopathology, ed 1. Amsterdam, Elsevier, 2004, pp 689–728.
7 Geomini P, Bremer G, Kruitwagen R, Mol BWJ: Diagnostic accuracy of frozen section diagnosis of the adnexal mass: a metaanalysis. Gynecol Oncol 2005;96:1–9.
8 Gol M, Baloglu A, Yigit S, Dogan Y, Aydin C, Yensel U: Accuracy of frozen section diagnosis in ovarian tumors: is there a change in the course of time? Int J Gynecol Cancer 2003;13:593–597.
9 Ilvan S. Ramazanoglu R, Akyldiz UE, Calay Z, Bese T, Oruc N: The accuracy of frozen section (intraoperative consultation) in the diagnosis of ovarian masses. Gynecol Oncol 2005;97:395–399.
10 Ittee S: Imprint cytologic examination as an adjunct to frozen section. J Med Assoc Thai 1993;76: 458–464.
11 Khunamornpong S, Siriaunkgul S: Scrape cytology of the ovaries: potential role in intraoperative consultation of ovarian lesions. Diagn cytopathol 2003;28:250–257.
12 Koss LG, Melamed MR: Tumors of the ovary and fallopian tube; in Koss L, Melamed M: Koss' Diagnostic Cytology and its Histopathologic Bases, ed 5. New York, Lippincott Williams & Wilkins, 2006, pp 491–508.
13 Malpica A. A SLAP. XXVI Congreso Latinoamericano de Patología. Punta del Este, 2007.
14 Michael CW, Lawrence WD, Bedrossian WM: Intraoperative consultation in ovarian lesions: a comparison between cytology and frozen section. Diagn Cytopathol 1996;15:387–394.
15 Nagai Y, Tanaka N, Horiuchi F, Ohki S, Seki K, Sekiya S: Diagnostic accuracy of intraoperative cytology in ovarian epithelial tumors. Int J Gynaecol Obstet 2001;72:159–164.
16 Pinto PB, Andrade L, Derchain S: Accuracy of intraoperative frozen section diagnosis of ovarian tumors. Gynecol Oncol 2001;81:230–232.
17 Prat J, Young RH: Selected Topics in Gynecologic Pathology. IAP 2006 Annual Congress. www.uscap.org/site/iap2006.
18 Robboy SJ, Mutter GL, Prat J, Bentley RC, Russell P, Anderson MC: Robboy's Pathology of the Female Reproductive Tract. Amsterdam, Elsevier, 2009, pp 729–778.
19 Saglam EA, Usubutun A, Ayhan A, Küçükali T: Mistakes prevent mistakes: experience for intraoperative consultation with frozen section. Gynecol Reprod Biol 2006;125:266–268.
20 Scucchi FL, Di Stefano D, Cosentino L, Vecchione A: Value of cytology as an adjuntive intraoperative diagnostic method: an audit of 2,250 consecutive cases. Acta Cytol 1997;41:1489–1496.
21 Seidman JD, Kurman RJ, Ronnet BM: Primary and metastatic mucinous adenocarcinomas in the ovaries: incidence in routine practice with a new approach to improve intraoperative diagnosis. Am J Surg Pathol 2003;27:985–993.
22 Shidham V: Role of scrape cytology in rapid intraoperative diagnosis: value and limitations. Acta Cytol 1984;28:477–482.
23 Shidham V, Galindo L, Edmonds P, George V: Intraoperative scrape cytology: comparison with frozen sections, using receiver, operating, characteristic (ROC) curve. Diagn Cytopathol 2000;23: 134–139.
24 Silva E: Frozen Section Of The Ovary. SAP 2005. Curso Internacional de Patología de la Sociedad Argentina de Patología. Buenos Aires, Argentina.
25 Souka S, Kamel M, Rocca M, El-Assi M, Hebeishy N, Sheir SH: The combined use of cytological imprint and frozen section in the intraoperative diagnosis of ovarian tumors. Int J Gynecol Obstet 1990;31:43–46.
26 Stewart Colin JR, Brennan BA, Hammond IG, Leung YC, McCartney AJ, et al: Intraoperative assessment of ovarian tumors: a 5-year review with assessment of discrepant diagnostic cases. Int J Gynecol Pathol 2006;25:216–222.
27 Tavassolli FA, Devilee P: Tumors of the Breast and Female Genital Organs. Lyon, IARC Press, 2003, pp 163–175.

Chapter 9

Glandular Lesions of the Vulva

The therapeutic results for malignant tumors of the vulva (3–4% of all malignant tumors of the female genital tract) are considerably worse than for the cervix, mainly due to major delays in the introduction and implementation of methods of prevention and early diagnosis, including cytodiagnosis. Two particularly important glandular lesions to be considered are vulvar Paget's disease (PD) and Bartholin's gland tumors, but there are several other less frequent lesions of special cytopathological interest, such as tumors of the specialized ano-genital mammary-like glands, the paraurethral (Skene) glands, minor vestibular glands, and tumors of skin appendage origin.

9.1. Histology of the Vulva

The external female genitalia include the mons pubis, labia majora and minora, the prepuce, frenulum, clitoris and vestibule. The orifices of the paraurethral (Skene) glands, of the major vestibular (Bartholin) glands and of the minor vestibular glands as well as the urethral meatus, open into the vestibule. The mons and labia majora are covered by keratinized, stratified squamous epithelium with hair follicles, sebaceous glands and sweat glands, including apocrine sweat glands. The epithelium of the labia minora is less keratinized, there are sebaceous and sweat glands but no hair follicles or underlying adipose tissue (fig. 9.1). The Skene's glands are composed of pseudostratified mucus-secreting columnar epithelium. The ducts are lined by transitional epithelium. The Bartholin's glands are tubulo-alveolar glands with acini composed of simple, columnar mucus-secreting epithelium. Their excretory ducts are lined by mucus-secreting epithelium proximally, transitional type epithelium distally and squamous epithelium at the opening. The minor vestibular glands are composed of acini lined by simple columnar mucus-secreting epithelium. There are also specialized ano-genital sweat glands (mammary-like) within the vulvar interlabial sulcus, medial aspects of the labia majora, perineum and around the anus. These glands are lined by simple columnar epithelium and myoepithelium.

9.2. Diagnosis of Vulvar Lesions

The prevention and early diagnosis of vulvar cancer is a challenge to gynecologists and pathologists, but also to women in general. Unfortunately, historically both patients and physicians have contributed to the delay in the early and

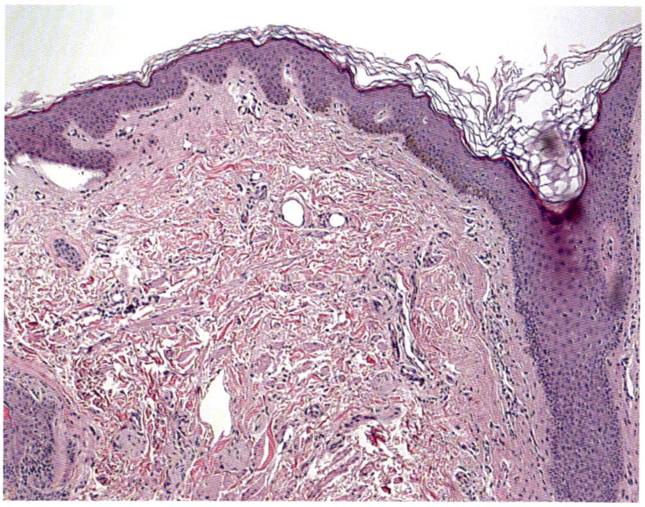

Fig. 9.1. Normal histology of the vulva.

accurate diagnosis of vulvar cancer. The delay is caused by patients failing to seek treatment for symptomatic lesions or chronic pruritus for between 2 and 16 months, while physicians often provide medical treatment of vulvar lesions for up to 12 months before proceeding to biopsy or referral [3].

Gynecological Examination. As a first step, routine annual visual inspection of the external genitals is recommended. This includes measurement of vulvar lesions, assessment of extension to adjacent structures, and bimanual pelvic examination. A thorough inspection of the perineal area and around the clitoris and urethra should be included. Palpation of the Bartholin's glands should also be performed. Neoplasia of the female genital is often multifocal. The vagina and cervix should be carefully inspected and a Pap-smear performed.

Vulvoscopy. Vulvoscopic examination should be the second step if any change is noted in the vulva or if there is persistent pruritus. 3–5% acetic must be applied for 3–5 min in advance, to allow for its absorption through the keratinized surface of the vulval skin. Colposcopic lesions can be classified as white, red and pigmented.

Cytology. Cytology material can be obtained from the vulva by the following methods: (1) Using wooden and metallic spatulas; (2) touching a glass slide directly against the lesion (note that both of these methods yield scanty material, and hyperkeratosis can cover deep tumors); (3) scraping with a scalpel blade after washing with saline (particularly in cases of hyperkeratosis, 2 or 3 scrapings may be necessary), and (4) fine needle aspiration of palpable subcutaneous or submucosal lesions of the vulva [13, 20]. We have been using the scalpel blade method since 1968. This gives the best results of the techniques described (fig. 9.2). Dennerstein, one of the pioneers of vulvar cytology, stated that poor results are mainly due to inadequate sampling and smear preparation techniques. Only scraping with a scalpel blade produces adequate smears suitable for diagnosis [6, 18].

Biopsy. Vulvar biopsy should be performed on all suspicious lesions, such as a confluent wart-like mass, a persistent pruritus, an ulcerated area, or when there has been a change in color of the surface of the lesion.

The vulvar biopsy is performed as an office procedure under local anesthesia, or by excision or punch biopsy. Excisional biopsy is preferred for lesions smaller than 1 cm in diameter.

A biopsy punch to the dermis is enough for a histological evaluation. It must include the surrounding skin with sufficient dermis and connective tissue to allow adequate pathological assessment of stromal invasion [3].

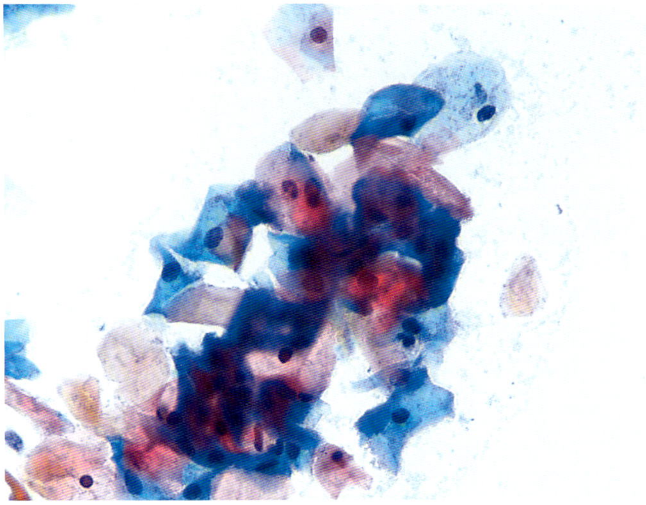

Fig. 9.2. Normal cytology of the vulva.

Complementary Explorations. Human papilomavirus (HPV) DNA detection can be applied, as HPV is a decisive factor in 20–50% of cases of invasive vulvar cancer. If a malignant tumor is diagnosed, we should determine how advanced the cancer is and how far it has spread. This includes measuring the size of the tumor and the depth of invasion into surrounding tissues and organs. Radiological imaging including a computed tomography scan can be used to assess the extent of the cancer. Endoscopic examination of the bladder (cystoscopy) and the rectum (protoscopy) may be performed if spread to these organs is suspected.

9.3. Concept of Vulvar Cancer

Malignant lesions of the vulva, the outer portion of the vagina, may be of epithelial (squamous and glandular) or mesenchymal (soft tissue) origin. Vulvar cancer is a rare type of neoplasm in women, 3–5% of all cancers of the female genital tract.

Epidemiology. Recent research [3] suggests that two different processes are involved in the development of vulvar cancer. The first type is vulvar intraepithelial neoplasia, caused mainly by HPV, with an increasing prevalence in young women. The second type is more common in older women and can develop from non-neoplastic epithelial vulvar lesions, following chronic inflammation. This is less frequent than the first type. High-risk HPV infection has been identified as an essential factor in the pathogenesis of vulvar cancer, although additional factors are necessary. DNA

Table 9.1. Cytologic terminology for vulvar descriptive diagnosis

1. Negative for intraepithelial lesion or malignancy
a. Organisms (vulvitis)
- trichomonas vaginalis
- shift in flora suggestive of bacterial vulvitis
- cellular changes consistent with herpes simplex virus

b. Other non-neoplastic findings (optional to report; list non-inclusive)
- reactive cellular changes associated with: inflammation, radiation, etc.
- atrophy

2. Other (see interpretation/result)

3. Epithelial cell abnormalities
Squamous cell
a. Vulvar atypical squamous cells
- of undetermined significance (VASC-US)
- cannot exclude VHSIL (VASC-H)

b. Vulvar squamous intraepithelial lesions (VSIL)
- low grade (VLSIL; encompassing HPV/mild dysplasia/VIN1, condyloma acuminatum)
- high grade [VHSIL; encompassing moderate dysplasia (VIN2), severe dysplasia and carcinoma in situ (VIN3)]

c. Squamous cell carcinoma

Glandular cell
a. Vulvar atypical glandular cells (VAGC)
b. Vulvar benign glandular cells: papillary hidradenoma
c. Vulvar malignant glandular cells: Paget disease, adenocarcinoma, etc.

VIN = Vulvar intraepithelial neoplasia.

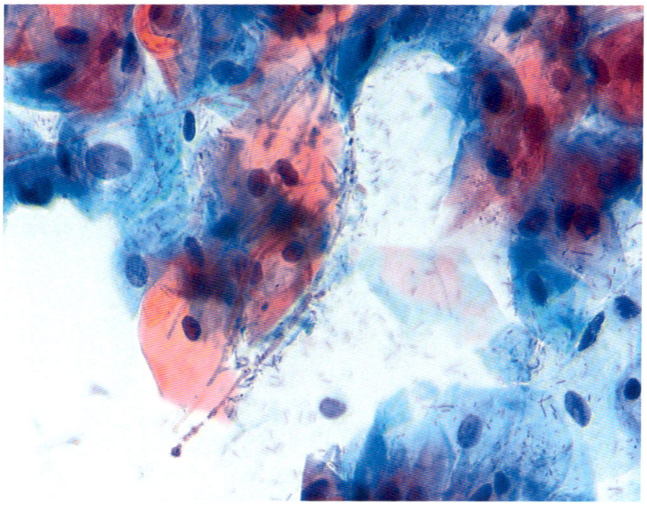

Fig. 9.3. Fungal vulvitis.

of a specific subtype of HPV (HPV_{16}) cannot be collected in up to 8% of vulvar cancers. Other viral antibodies, such as herpes virus type 2, are independent risk factors. Finally, factors that play an important role in the development of endometrial adenocarcinoma, such as hypertension, diabetes and obesity, have been found at most in 25% of vulvar cancers [3].

Clinical Features. The most frequent symptom of vulvar cancer is an enduring pruritus. Other major symptoms are pain and bleeding unrelated to the menstrual cycle. During the menstrual cycle the skin of the vulva oscillates between white and rough. On physical examination the vulvar cancerous growth may appear fleshy, ulcerated, leukoplakic or verrucous. The most frequent locations for vulvar cancer are the labia majora and minora.

Diagnosis. Vulvar screening should be included in the annual genital examination as mentioned.

The gold standard for the diagnosis of vulvar tumor is the biopsy, which is indicated in any suspected lesions, including wart-like growth, persistent pruritus, ulcerated areas or changes in the color, growth or surface of a lesion [3].

9.4. Terminology for Reporting Vulvar Cytology

In 1997 we introduced a new terminology for vulvar cytology based on the Bethesda System [22] and WHO Classification [23], which was presented for the first time at the IAC Conference in Kamuela, Hawai, in 1997 [13]. The following elements of vulvar cytology were recommended for reporting: adequacy of specimen, general categorization and descriptive diagnosis. The terminology of vulvar lesions includes benign cellular changes (vulvitis and reactives changes) and epithelial cell abnormalities [14] (table 9.1).

General Categorization (Optional). This element has been changed following the new categories at Bethesda 2001: (1) negative for intraepithelial lesion or malignancy; (2) other (see 'Interpretation/Result'), and (3) epithelial cell abnormalities.

Interpretation/Result. As in cervical cytology the term diagnosis has been replaced by interpretation or result.

Organisms. Vulvar cytology permits reporting of trichomonas vaginalis, fungal organisms (fig. 9.3) and herpes simplex virus (fig. 9.4).

Other Non-Neoplastic Findings. Reactive cellular changes associated with inflammation, radiation, etc., or atrophy.

Epithelial Cell Abnormalities. These include squamous and glandular cell abnormalities. As in the 2001 Bethesda

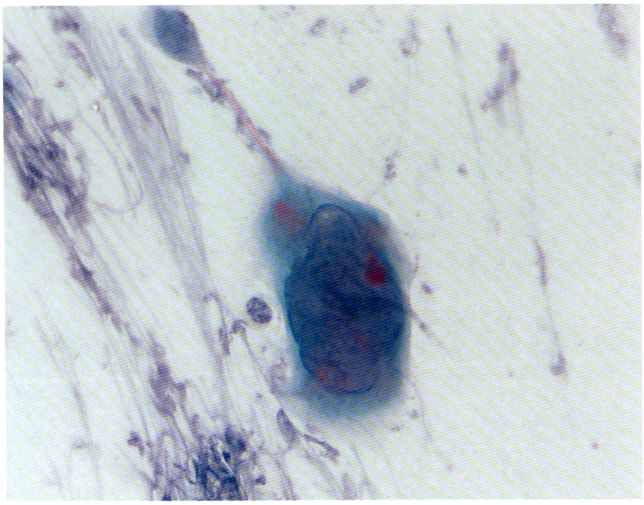

Fig. 9.4. Herpes simplex virus.

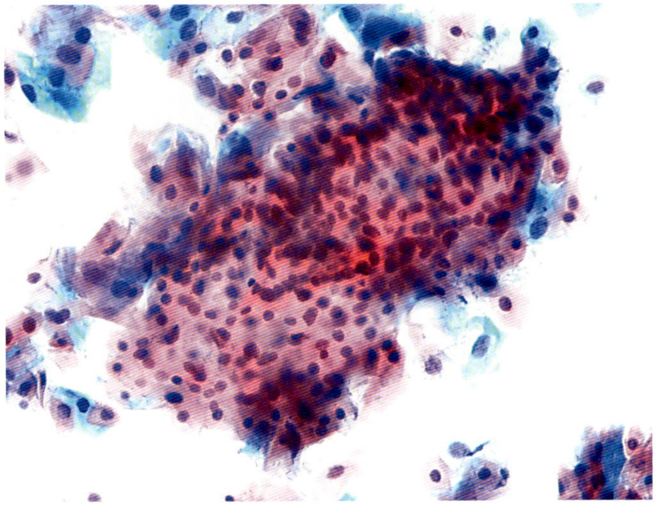

Fig. 9.6. Vulvar high grade SIL.

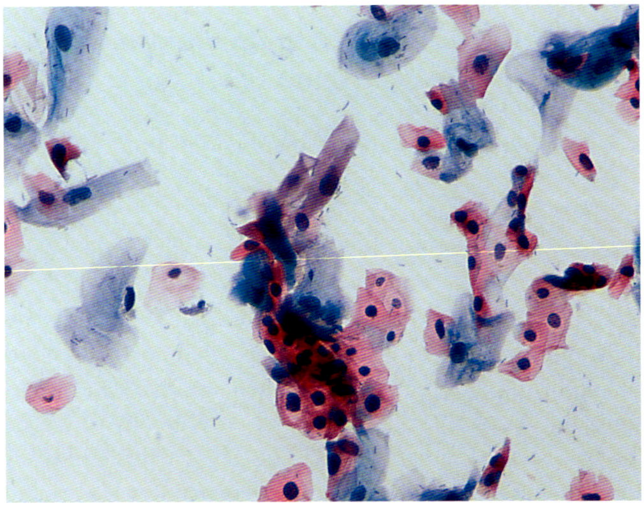

Fig. 9.5. Vulvar low grade SIL.

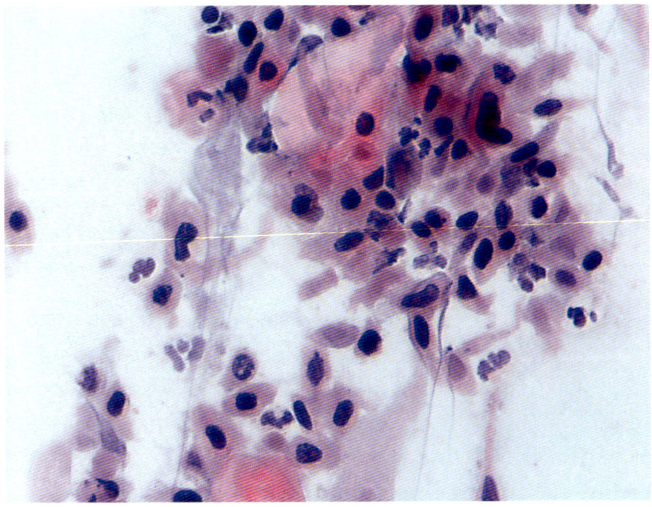

Fig. 9.7. Vulvar squamous cell carcinoma.

Sytem, squamous cell abnormalities can be divided into vulvar atypical squamous cells, vulvar low-grade squamous intraepithelial lesion (SIL; fig. 9.5), vulvar high-grade SIL (fig. 9.6) and squamous cell carcinoma (fig. 9.7). The glandular cell abnormalites can be divided into atypical glandular cells, vulvar benign glandular cells and vulvar malignant glandular cells. The most common glandular tumors are papillary hidradenoma, PD, adenocarcinoma of Bartholin's glands and secondary tumors (table 9.2).

9.5. Cytopathology of Glandular Tumors of the Vulva

9.5.1. Paget Disease

This is a form of in situ adenocarcinoma of the squamous mucosa that shows apocrine or eccrine glandular-like features. The origin of vulvar PD is controversial. There are 2 possibilities:

- Cutaneous origin. Pluripotential stem cell within the epidermis, or in situ malignant transformation of cells in the epidermal sweat ducts.

Table 9.2. WHO histological classification of glandular tumors of the vulva

Paget disease
Bartholin gland tumors
Adenocarcinoma
Squamous cell carcinoma
Adenoid cystic carcinoma
Adenosquamous carcinoma
Transitional cell carcinoma
Small cell carcinoma
Adenoma
Adenomyoma
Others
Tumors arising from specialized anogenital mammary-like glands
Adenocarcinoma of mammary gland type
Papillary hidradenoma
Others
Adenocarcinoma of Skene gland origin
Adenocarcinomas of other types
Adenoma of minor vestibular glands
Mixed tumor of the vulva
Tumors of skin appendage origin
Malignant sweat gland tumors
Sebaceous carcinoma
Syringoma
Nodular hidradenoma
Trichoepithelioma
Trichilemmoma
Others
Secondary tumors

- Underlying skin appendage adenocarcinoma, ano-rectal or urothelial carcinoma.

In 10–20% of cases PD is associated with an underlying invasive adenocarcinoma arising from the vulvar glands, Bartholin's or sweat glands.

Epidemology. Primary cutaneous PD is an uncommon tumor; most cases occur in postmenopausal white women. The average age at presentation is 67 years.

Clinical Features. The findings are usually an eczematoid lesion that clinically resembles a dermatitis, which may delay the diagnosis. The labia majora are the most frequently involved sites. The prognosis depends on the presence of an invasive carcinoma (10–20% of cases) and on the extent of the disease.

Histopathology. This intraepithelial lesion is characterized by the presence of Paget cells in an acanthotic squamous epithelium, including the granular and keratin layers (fig. 9.8). The Paget cells are large, round cells with a large nucleus, prominent nucleolus, and a pale and often vacuolated cytoplasm. They contain abundant mucin, which can be confirmed by mucicarmine, alcian blue (pH 2.5), colloidal iron and PAS stains. With immunohistochemical techniques the Paget cells stain positive for carcinoembryonic antigen, low-molecular-weight cytokeratins and epithelial membrane antigen. They are negative for CD44 or S100 protein and have the immunophenotype CK7+/CK20–. These markers are useful for distinguishing PD from Bowen's disease or melanoma in situ.

Cytology. Paget cells are found as single cells or clusters of cells in cytological smears. They are large, with variable amounts of cytoplasm. The nuclei are enlarged, usually eccentric and with nucleoli (fig. 9.9). Occasional signet-ring

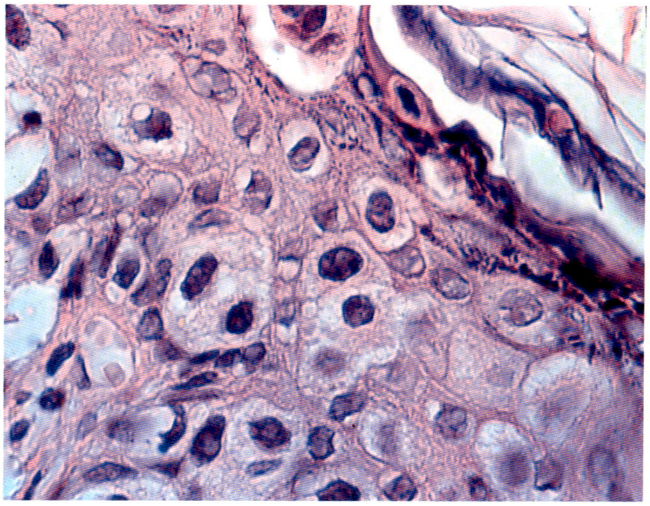

Fig. 9.8. Histology of vulvar Paget disease.

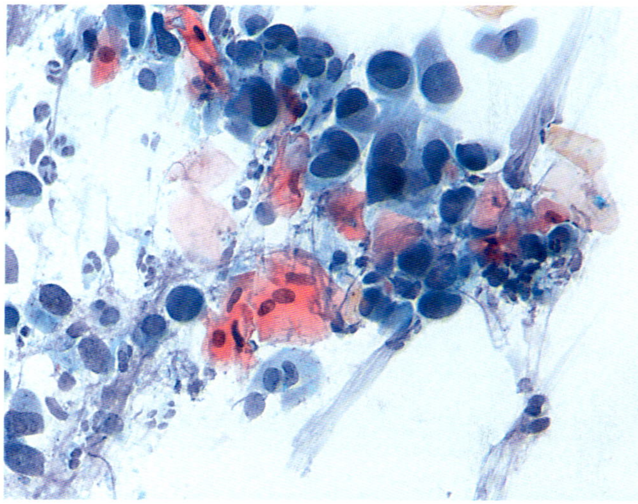

Fig. 9.9. Cytology of vulvar Paget disease.

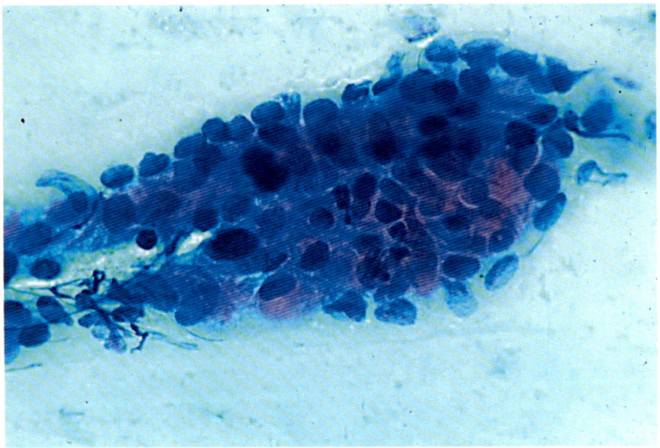

Fig. 9.10. FNA cytology of a Bartholin gland adenocarcinoma.

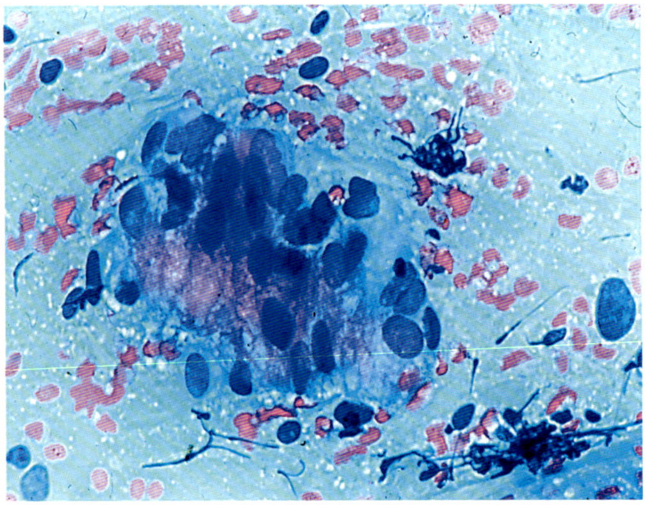

Fig. 9.11. FNA cytology of a Bartholin gland adenocarcinoma.

forms are observed [2]. In rare cases, PD can extend to the vagina and cervix and can be diagnosed in a cervicovaginal smear [10]. Cytological examination by scraping with a scalpel blade is useful in the follow-up after surgical excision, due to the high recurrence rate [9].

Differential Diagnosis. The differential diagnosis of extramammary PD is primary adenocarcinoma arising from vulvar glands or from the Batholin's glands, and tumors of the ano-genital mammary-like glands. Tumors metastatic to the vulva should also be included. In most cases of PD, typical Paget cells are not difficult to find due to their isolated arrangement and rounded appearance, contrasting with the glandular malignant cells in cases of adenocarcinoma. PD

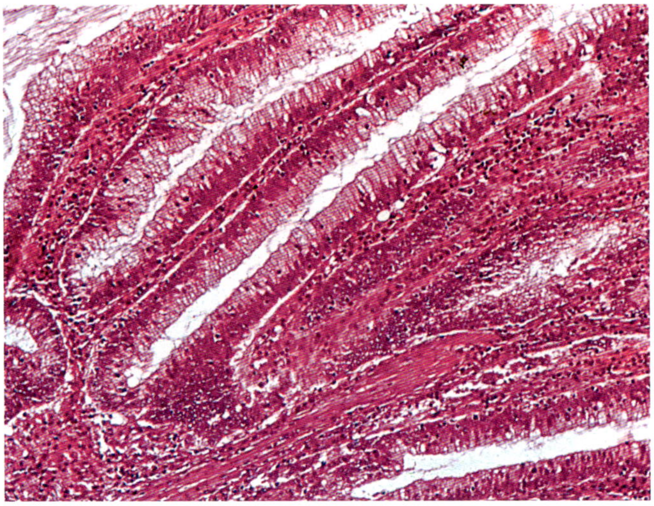

Fig. 9.12. Histology of a Bartholin gland adenocarcinoma.

must also be differentiated from Bowen's disease and melanoma in situ.

9.5.2. Bartholin Gland Carcinoma

Primary carcinoma of diverse cells types located in the site of the Bartholin's glands. Bartholin gland carcinoma (BGC) is an uncommon neoplasia that occurs predominantly in women over 50 years of age. The symptoms and signs are not specific and may include pain, swelling, dyspareunia and pruritus [9]. Clinical examination reveals an enlargement in the Bartholin's glands area that may resemble a Batholin's duct cyst.

Histopathology. The BGC is a typically solid and deeply infiltrative tumor. Various types with glandular malignant patterns have been described:

- Adenocarcinoma accounts for approximately 40% of Bartholin's gland tumors. Adenocarcinomas may be mucinous, papillary or mucoepidermoid in type [12] (fig. 9.10–9.12).
- Adenoid cystic carcinoma accounts for 15% of Bartholin's gland tumors. It is composed of rounded islands of uniform malignant epithelial cells with a cribriform pattern. A hyaline stroma may form cylinders separating rows of tumor cells (fig. 9.13).
- Adenosquamous carcinoma is composed of neoplastic mucin-containing glandular cells and neoplastic squamous cells.

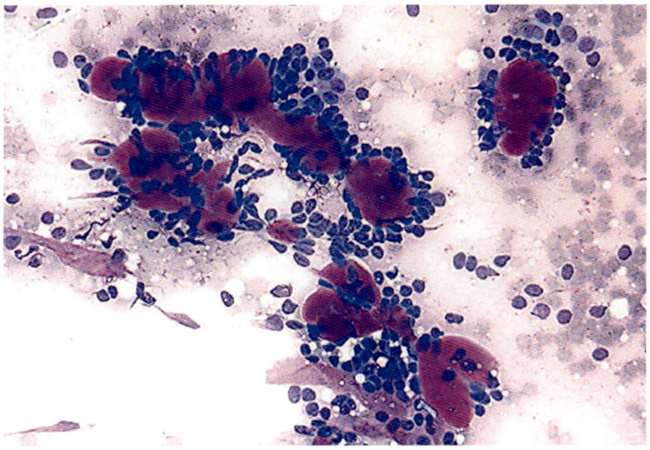

Fig. 9.13. FNA of an adenoid cystic carcinoma of the Bartholin gland.

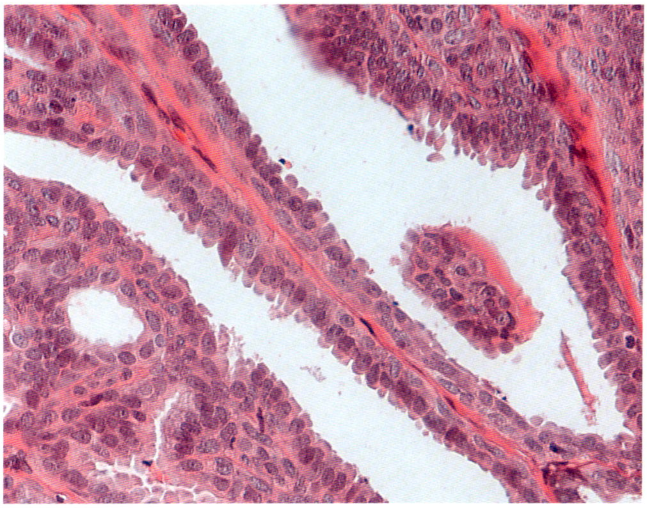

Fig. 9.14. Histology of a papillary hidradenoma of the vulva.

- Other carcinomas. There are also pure squamous cell carcinomas (40% of Bartholin gland tumors), transitional cell carcinomas and small cell carcinomas.

Cytology. Because none of the cell types are unique for BGC, the cytological and histological patterns correlate.

Diagnosis. The diagnosis of BGC is usually made by biopsy. Cytological examination may help to avoid delay in the diagnosis.

Differential Diagnosis. Although a cytological diagnosis may not always be possible due to a deep location of BGC, this tumor should be considered in the differential diagnosis when malignant cells are identified in smears and no upper genital tract lesions are found [5].

9.5.3. Tumors Arising from Specialized Anogenital Mammary-Like Glands

Malignant and benign tumors, usually of glandular type and resembling neoplasms of the breast, may arise in specialized anogenital mammary-like glands. These glands and the tumors that arise from them are usually identified in or adjacent to the intralabial sulcus.

9.5.3.1. Papillary Hidradenoma

Papillary hidradenoma (PH) is a benign tumor composed of epithelial secretory cells and underlying myoepithelial cells lining complex branching papillae with delicate fibrovascular cores.

Clinical Features. PH is the most common benign glandular neoplasm. The lesion is small and in most cases asymptomatic. However, it may cause bleeding mimicking carcinoma if the gland has prolapsed and/or ulcerated. It usually does not require excision. PH develops in labia majora, labia minora and the interlabial sulci of the vulva. It rarely appears in the perineum and perianal region [19].

Histopathology. It presents as a solitary, round, firm, dome-shaped lesion of 2–3 cm diameter. It may ulcerate, giving rise to a fungating red tumor, which tends to bleed. The tumor is intradermal, well circumscribed and has a tubular and papillary growth pattern. The tubules and acini are lined by a single or double layer of columnar cells with underlying smaller myoepithelial cells (fig. 9.14).

Cytology. PH presents 3 types of cells: columnar, myoepithelial and metaplastic apocrine cells. Clumps of slightly pleomorphic glandular cells are seen with a fine, evenly distributed chromatin. The cellular arrangement and the N/C ratio are evidence of its benign nature (fig. 9.15). The appearance of the cytological smear resembles that of an endocervical polyp [1, 7, 11, 21].

Differential Diagnosis. The differential diagnosis of PH must include extra mammary PD, a rare primary adenocarcinoma arising either in the sweat glands of the labia or in the Bartholin's glands, and adenocarcinoma metastatic from another site. Paget cells are readily identified by their single-cell arrangement and rounded appearance.

An erroneous diagnosis of adenocarcinoma is possible on microscopic examination, but cells from an adenocarcinoma should have obvious malignant features. A careful study of the histological specimen together with cytological and colposcopic examination may be necessary. We believe that both diagnostic tools, as is universally accepted for the

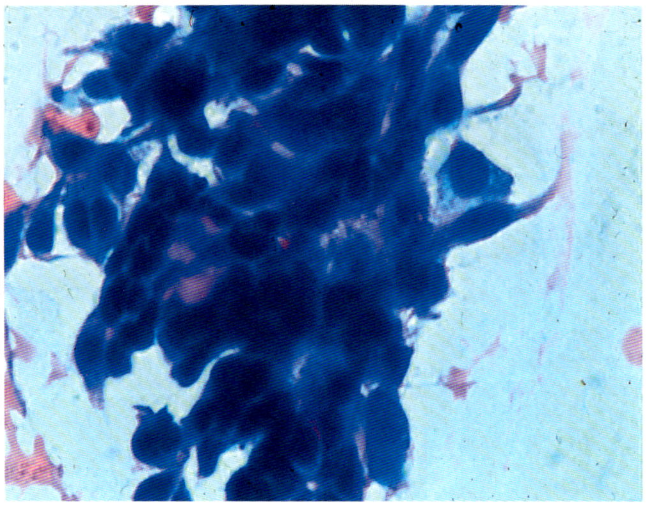

Fig. 9.15. FNA cytology of a papillary hidradenoma of the vulva.

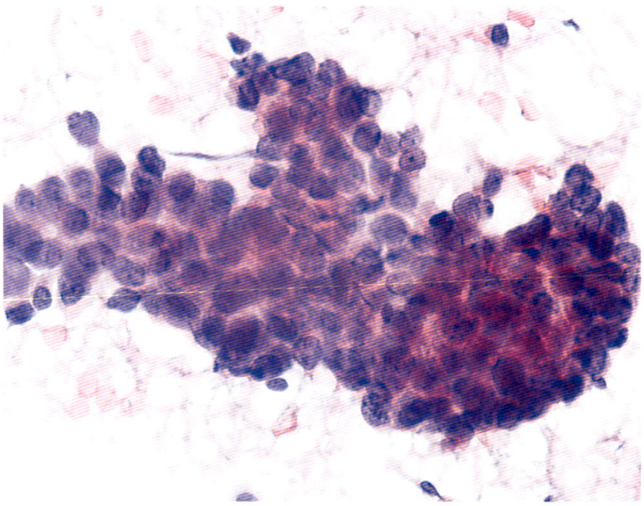

Fig. 9.16. FNA cytology of an adenocarcinoma arising from specialized anogenital mammary-like glands.

prevention and early diagnosis of cervical tumors, should be applied in the diagnosis of benign and malignant lesions of the vulva [15, 16].

9.5.3.2. Adenocarcinomas and Other Tumors Arising from Specialized Anogenital Mammary-Like Glands

Carcinoma resembling breast carcinoma, mostly of the infiltrating ductal type, as well as benign (fibroadenoma), Phyllodes [4] and other malignant tumors of mammary type rarely arise in ectopic breast tissue (fig. 9.16). A case

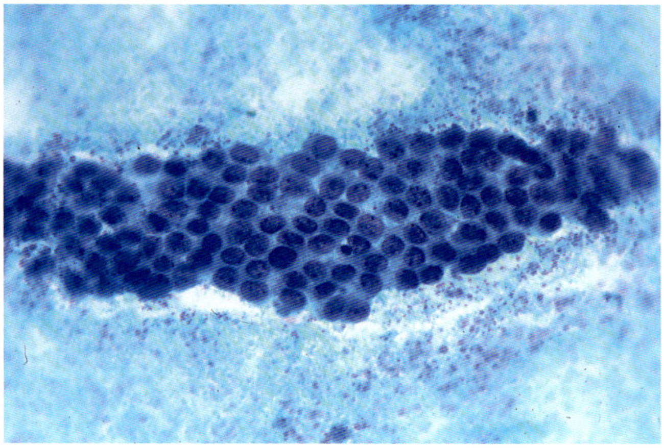

Fig. 9.17. FNA cytology of a Bartholin cyst gland.

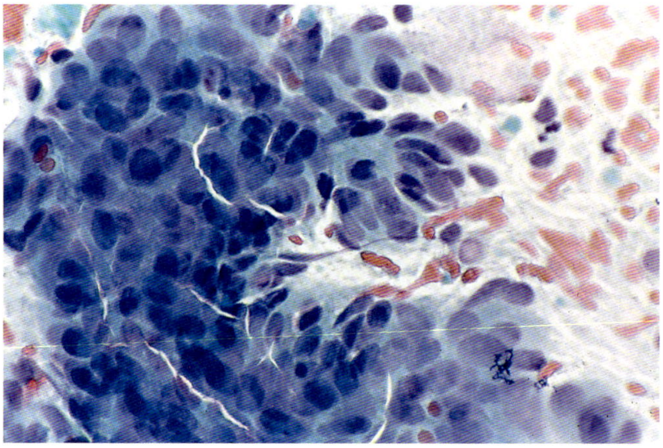

Fig. 9.18. FNA cytology of a metastatic vulvar tumor from an endometrial adenocarcinoma.

Table 9.3. Cytodiagnosis of vulvar lesions

Cytodiagnosis	Cases, n	%
Normal vulva	132	23.46
Vulvitis	220	39.09
VSIL	141	25.06
Condyloma acuminatum	4	0.71
Lymphocytic leukemia	1	0.17
Squamous cell carcinoma	56	9.94
Bartholin's adenocarcinoma	1	0.17
Postirradiation	1	0.17
Vulvar cyst	1	0.17
Unsatisfactory	6	1.06
Total	*563*	*100.00*

VSIL = Vulvar squamous intraepithelial lesions.

of adenocarcinoma in situ of breast tissue associated with a vulvar papillary hidradenoma has recently been published, suggesting a close relationship between papillary hidradenoma and breast tissue [20].

9.5.4. Other Benign Tumors

Bartholin cyst gland (fig. 9.17), adenoma and adenomyoma of the Bartholin gland, and adenoma of minor vestibular glands are rare benign tumors. Mixed tumor of the vulva (pleomorphic adenoma) is composed of epithelial cells arranged in tubules or nests mixed with a fibromyxoid stroma with chondroid or osseus elements. Finally, benign tumors of skin appendage origin differentiating towards hair follicles, sweat or sebaceous glands, such as syringoma, nodular hidradenoma, trichoepithelioma and trichilemmoma, should also be mentioned.

9.5.5. Other Malignant Tumors

Adenocarcinomas may arise from the glands of Skene (they express prostatic antigen [22]), or from skin appendages, including carcinoma of sweat gland origin (eccrine adenocarcinoma, porocarcinoma, hidradenocarcinoma and apocrine adenocarcinoma, the last of which may be associated with PD) and sebaceous carcinomas.

9.5.6. Secondary Tumors

Metastatic spread to the vulva from tumors of the endometrium (fig. 9.18), ovary, cervix, breast, gastrointestinal tract, urethra and lymphoma have been reported.

9.6. Cytodiagnosis of Vulvar Lesions

Personal Experience. The results of the Cytology Laboratory of the Hospital Universitario Gregorio Marañón of Madrid up to 2001 have been reported [15]. The number of cytological diagnoses of vulvar lesions and the percentage of each diagnosis are shown in table 9.3. Among 563 cases, the diagnoses were normal vulva (23.46%), vulvitis (39.09%), vulvar squamous intraepithelial lesions (25.06%), condyloma acuminatum (0.71%) and squamous cell carinoma (9.94%). Six cases (1.06%) were unsatisfactory for evaluation. Histological examination was performed in 147 patients (26.11%), and the cyto-histologic correlation is shown in table 9.4. Among 57 cytologic diagnoses of malignancy there was 1 false positive and no false negative reports. The level of accuracy was high, as shown in table 9.5.

Table 9.4. Cytodiagnosis of vulvar lesions: cytohistologic correlations

Cytodiagnosis	Histological diagnosis										Total	%
	Normal	Vulvitis	VSIL	Condyloma	Papilloma	Hematoma	Hidradenoma	Cancer	Leukemia	Batholin's gland abscess		
Normal vulva	4	6	9				1				20	13.60
Vulvitis		5	2		1						8	5.44
Cocci vulvitis		9	4	1	2						16	10.88
Fungal vulvitis		1									1	0.68
Atrophic vulvitis		2									2	1.36
Gardnerella		1									1	0.68
VSIL	5	6	20		1	1	1	2			36	24.49
Condyloma				3				1			4	2.72
Squamous cell carcinoma			1					53			54	36.75
Lymphoma/ leukemia									1		1	0.68
Bartholin's adenocarcinoma										1	1	0.68
Unsatisfactory	1		1	1							3	2.04
Total	*10*	*30*	*37*	*5*	*4*	*1*	*2*	*56*	*1*	*1*	*147*	*100.00*

VSIL = Vulvar squamous intraepithelial lesions

Table 9.5. Vulvar cytology accuracy

Diagnosis	Sensitivity, %	Specificity, %
Benign	96.70	98.87
Malignant	98.21	94.82

Advantages of Vulvar Cytodiagnosis. Vulvar cytodiagnosis offers a complete evaluation of the vulvar epithelium, in contrast to biopsy, which evaluates only small atypical areas. It is painless and easy to repeat. It also has a high accuracy in the diagnosis of benign and malignant cases. Furthermore, it indicates the most appropriate areas for biopsies.

Indication for Vulvar Cytodiagnosis. Vulvar cytodiagnosis is preventive in women over 50 years of age, in association with other preventive techniques. Vulvar cytodiagnosis is useful for all vulvar lesions, both clinically benign and malignant, especially vulvar dystrophies. It is also useful in the follow-up of dystrophies and after therapy for neoplasms.

9.7. Final Remarks

Vulvar cytodiagnosis allows reporting on the type of vulvar lesions, infections and inflammatory diseases included, and is an important method in the detection of cancer and its precursors. Its use shortens the delay in the diagnosis of vulvar cancer.

References

1 Abdul-Karim T, Somrak TM, Young B: Vulva, vagina and anus; in Bibbo M, Wilbur DC (eds): Compressive Cytopathology, ed 3. Amsterdam, Elselvier, 2008, pp 273–289.

2 Bennington JL, Smith DC, Figge DC: Detection of cells from extramammary Paget's disease of the vulva in a vaginal smear: report of a case. Obstet Gynecol 1996;27:772–775.

3 Canavan TB, Cohen D: Vulvar cancer. Am Fam Physician 2002;66:1269–1274.

4 Chulia MT, Paya A, Niveiro M, Ceballos S, Aranda FI: Phyllodes tumor in ectopic breast tissue of the vulva. Int J Surg Pathol 2001;91:81–83.

5 De Mauro JM, Skolom J, Wallach RC, Rorat E: Cytologic diagnosis of Bartholin's gland adenocarcinoma. Acta Cytol 1986;30:491–493.

6 Dennerstein GJ: The cytology of the vulva. J Obstet Gynaecol Br Commonw 1968;75:603–609.

7 Duppie-Froment J: Cytologie gynécologique. Paris, Flamarion, 1974, p 41.

8 Fanning J, Lambert HC, Hale TM, Morris PC, Schuerch C: Paget's disease of the vulva: prevalence of associated vulvar adenocarcinoma, invasive Paget's disease, and recurrence after surgical excision. Am J Obstet Gynecol 1999;180:24–27.

9 Felix JC, Cote RJ, Kramen EE, Saigo P, Goldman GH: Carcinoma of the Bartholin's gland: histogenesis and the ethiological role of human papilloma virus. Am J Pathol 1993;142:925–933.

10 Gu M, Ghafari S, Lin F: Pap smears of patients with extramammary Paget's disease of the vulva. Diagn Cytopathol 2005;32:353–357.

11 Hustin J, Donnay M, Hamels J: Identification of papillary hidradenoma of the vulva by imprint cytology. Acta Cytol 1980;24:466–467.

12 Imachi M, Tsukamoto N, Shigematsu T, Nakano H: Cytologic diagnosis of primary adenocarcinoma of Bartholin's gland: a case report. Acta Cytol 1992; 36:167–170.

13 Jiménez-Ayala M: Cytologic terminology of the vulva: report of the task force on terminology. Diagnostic cytology towards the 21st century. An International expert conference and tutorial. Kamuela, 1997.

14 Jiménez-Ayala M, Jiménez-Ayala B: Terminology for vulvar cytology based on the Bethesda System. Acta Cytol 2002;46:645–650.

15 Jiménez-Ayala M, Vilaplana E, Nogales OF, Nogales FF: Citología Ginecológica. Second edition. Barcelona, Ed Científico Médica, 1985, pp 99–115.

16 Jiménez-Ayala M, Vilaplana E, Pereira A, Pérez-Barroso M, Granados M, Saiz-Pardo FS, Alvarez J: Cytodiagnostique des lésions vulvaires. Arch Anat Cytol Pathol 1976;24:339–345.

17 Kurman RJ, Solomon D: The Bethesda System for reporting cervical/vaginal cytologic diagnosis. New York, Springer, 1994, pp 3–60.

18 Nauth MF, Boger A: New aspects of vulvar cytology. Acta Cytol 1982;26:1–6.

19 Rolling SD: Fine-needle aspiration diagnosis of a vulvar papillary hidradenoma: a case report. Diagn Cytopathol 1994;10:60–61.

20 Shah SS, Adelson M, Mazur MT: Adenocarcinoma in situ arising in vulvar papillary hidradenoma: report of 2 cases. Int J Gynecol Pathol 2008;27:453–456.

21 Schramm G: Diagnosis of a papillary hidradenoma of the vulva by simultaneous cytology and colposcopy. Acta Cytol 1979;23:57–60.

22 Solomon D, Nayar R (eds): The Bethesda System for reporting cervical cytology, ed 2. New York, Springer, 2004.

23 Wilkinson EJ, Teixeira MR: Tumors of the vulva: epithelial tumors; in Fattaneh A, Tavassoli FA, Devilee P: Tumors of the breast and female genital tract. Lyon, IARC Press, 2003, pp 314–330.

Chapter 10

Glandular Lesions of the Fallopian Tube

10.1. Histology of the Fallopian Tube

The fallopian tubes (FT) are paired, tubular, seromuscular organs that extend from the cornua of the uterus toward the corresponding ovary. The tubes are situated at the upper margins of the broad ligaments between the round and utero-ovarian ligaments. The abdominal ostium is situated at the base of the infundibulum, the circumference of which is enhanced by irregular processes called fimbriae. The infundibulum narrows gradually and merges with the ampullary portion of the tube. It continues as the isthmus and the interstitial or corneal portion of the tube.

The tubal wall consists of 3 layers: the internal mucosa (endosalpinx), the intermediate muscular layer (myosalpinx), and the outer serosa, which is continuous with the peritoneum of the broad ligament and uterus. The endosalpinx is thrown into longitudinal folds, lined by columnar epithelium of 3 types: ciliated, secretory, and intercalary cells. There are scattered lymphocytes located basally above the basement membrane (fig. 10.1).

The tubal muscularis generally has 2 layers: an outer longitudinal layer and an inner circular layer.

The serosa of the tube is composed of a mesothelial layer histologically indistinguishable from the peritoneum.

Wolffian or mesonephric duct remnants are commonly found on routine sections. The tubules are lined by ciliated and non-ciliated cuboidal or low columnar cells.

10.2. Benign Fallopian Tube Lesions

Metaplasia. This presents as an abrupt transition between normal tubal and mucinous epithelium. The mucinous epithelium shows no evidence of invasion or destruction of the lamina propia or myosalpinx. Mucinous metaplasia of the FT may be a marker for multiple mucinous neoplasia. It can be associated with Peutz-Jeghers syndrome.

Endometriosis. This is an ectopic presence of endometrial tissue with stroma and glands within a fibrotic tissue that may replace normal tubal epithelium and cause luminal occlusion.

Endosalpingiosis. This is a benign transformation of the mesothelium into tubal epithelium, with ciliated and secretory cells.

10.3. Tumors of the Fallopian Tube

The WHO Histological Classification of the epithelial tumors of the FT is presented in table 10.1 [1].

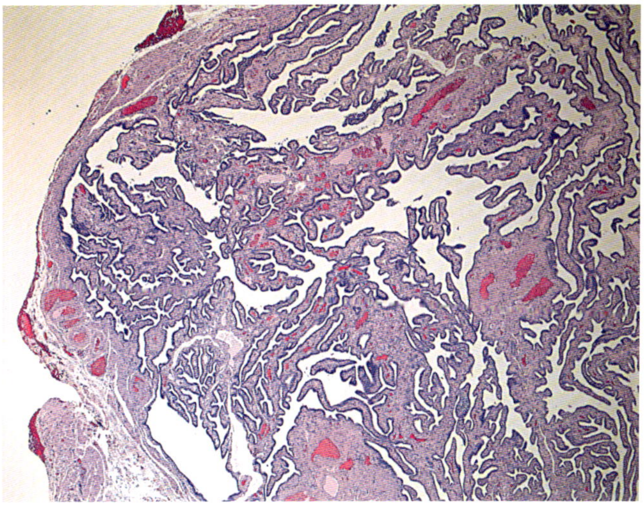

Fig. 10.1. Histology of a normal fallopian tube.

Table 10.1. WHO Histological Classification of tumors of the fallopian tube (2003)

1. Epithelial tumors
   - Malignant tumors
     - Serous adenocarcinoma
     - Mucinous adenocarcinoma
     - Endometrioid adenocarcinoma
     - Clear cell adenocarcinoma
     - Transitional cell carcinoma
     - Squamous cell carcinoma
     - Undifferentiated carcinoma
     - Others
   - Borderline tumors (of low malignant potential)
     - Serous borderline tumor
     - Mucinous borderline tumor
     - Endometrioid borderline tumor
     - Others
   - Carcinoma in situ
   - Benign tumors
     - Papilloma (specify type)
     - Cystadenofibroma (specify type)
     - Metaplastic papillary tumor
     - Endometrioid polyp
     - Others
2. Mixed epithelial-mesenchymal tumors
3. Soft tissue tumors
4. Mesothelial tumors
5. Germ cell tumors
6. Trophoblastic disease
7. Lymphoid and hematopoietic tumors
8. Secondary tumors

10.3.1. Benign Epithelial Tumors

Benign epithelial tubal neoplasms are rare and include papillomas, serous or mucinous cystadenomas, adenofibromas and cystadenofibromas, metaplastic papillary tumors and endometrial (adenomatous) polyps.

10.3.2. Malignant Epithelial Tumors

Malignant neoplasms of the fallopian tube are the rarest of the gynecologic cancers. While cancers metastatic to the FT occur frequently from ovary, endometrium, or other sources, and while there are reports of transitional cell carcinoma, adenosquamous carcinomas, and sarcomas, almost all of the primary cancers of the fallopian tube are papillary adenocarcinomas [4].

The criteria to establish primary fallopian tube cancer were laid down by Hu and colleagues [12] and later modified slightly by Sedlis [16]:

- Grossly: the main tumor is in the tube and arises from the endosalpinx.
- Histologically: the pattern reproduces the epithelium of tubal mucosa (papillary pattern).
- Transition from benign to malignant tubal epithelium should be demonstrated.
- The ovaries and endometrium are normal or have a much smaller tumor volume than that of the tube.

Clinical Features. Primary fallopian tube carcinoma (FTC) is rare, accounting for 0.3–1.1% of gynecological malignancies, and is more frequent in infertile and postmenopausal women. Incidence peaks between 60 and 64 years of age, and then declines until 84 years [4].

The incidence rate in the USA – calculated on the basis of 3,051 primary FTC diagnosed between 1998 and 2003 – is 0.4 per 100,000 women. White, non-hispanic women and women age 60–79 have the highest incidence rates [19]. There is evidence that individuals with mutations of BRCA1 and BRCA2 are at higher risk for the development of FTC.

The most frequent symptoms are vaginal bleeding, unexplained serosanguineous vaginal discharge and pelvic pain. Uterine bleeding is almost always unexplained by uterine curettage [9]. The pain is highly significant since cancer of the ovary, endometrium, and cervix do not cause pain until the diagnosis is already obvious. The syndrome 'hydrops tubae profluens', with profuse vaginal discharge, is almost pathognomonic, but infrequent. Risk factors appear similar to those of epithelial ovarian cancer. The tumor is usually discovered late and has a poor prognosis [2, 9].

Histopathology. FTC presents the same histological subtypes as ovarian carcinoma (table 10.1).

The most common type is serous adenocarcinoma. In the largest series of 3,051 cases [19], 88% of were in this category, half of the cases were poorly differentiated and 89% were unilateral at diagnosis. Overall rates of FTC remained stable overtime. Although the demographic characteristics of FTC are similar to those of ovarian cancers; stage at diagnosis and the stable trend observed in FTC are in contrast to ovarian cancer.

The other tumor types include mucinous, endometrioid, clear cell adenocarcinoma, transitional cell carcinoma, undifferentiated carcinoma, and mixed types.

Serous Adenocarcinoma. Serous tumors are graded with respect to their differentiation and extent of solid components: most tumors are invasive tumors poorly differentiated (fig. 10.2) [8].

Mucinous Adenocarcinoma. These tumors are extremely rare and are often associated with other mucinous neoplasms

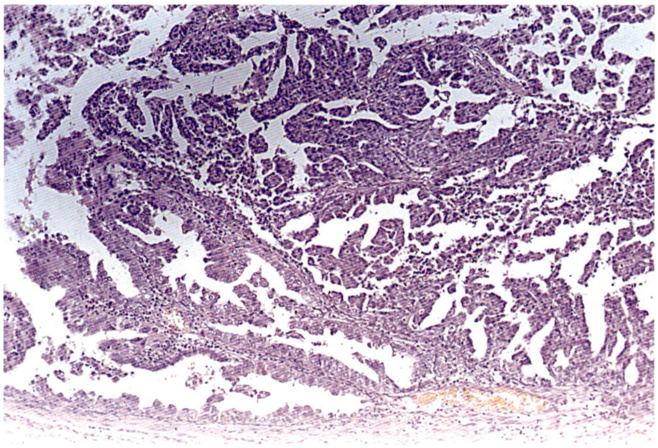

Fig. 10.2. Serous adenocarcinoma of the fallopian tube.

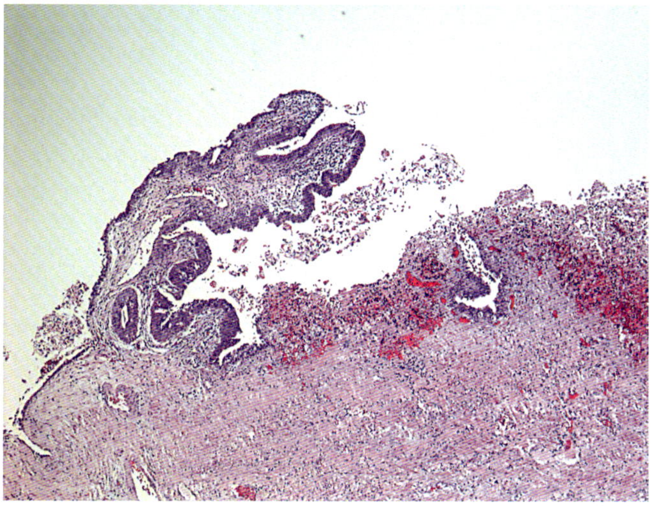

Fig. 10.3. Carcinoma in situ of the fallopian tube.

of the genital tract, including trifocal MA [13]. Most cases are in situ mucinous carcinomas. The histological features of tubal MA are similar to those of the ovarian counterpart. Goblet cells may be predominant [17].

Endometrioid adenocarcinoma of the FT. This is characteristically non-invasive or only superficially invasive and has a good prognosis. The tumor closely resembles its uterine counterpart [1]. A few cases of endometrioid adenocarcinoma of the FT resembling an adnexal tumor of probable Wolfian origin have been published [6, 7]. Microscopically, the tumors are characterized by a predominant pattern of small, closely packed cells, surrounded by numerous glandular spaces. Concentric whorls of spindle cells may be seen in the solid areas in some cases. A large number of cases of endometrioid adenocarcinoma simultaneously involving the uterus and the FT have been published by the Anderson Cancer Center [5]. FT involvement could be explained as a luminal extension of the endometrial carcinoma.

Clear Cell Carcinoma. This type of tubal carcinoma shows a tubulocystic pattern with prominent hobnail and clear cells.

10.3.3. Borderline Epithelial Tumors

Borderline epithelial tumors of the FT are rare and include cases of serous, mucinous and endometrioid types.

10.3.4. Carcinoma in situ

The diagnosis of early primary tubal cancer is difficult. In situ and early invasive carcinomas of the FT have usually found incidentally.

Carcinoma in situ shows replacement of the tubal epithelium by malignant glandular cells with pleomorphic nuclei (fig 10.3).

Rare cases of carcinoma in situ of the FT have been described showing adenocarcinoma cells in a Pap-smear or in an endometrial smear [15]. Cytologic examination obtained by hydrotubation may be useful in diagnosing early tubal cancer.

10.4. Diagnosis of Tubal Carcinoma

Preoperative diagnosis of FT malignancy is very difficult, especially in the early stages, and is only made in less of 10% of cases [3].

Pelvic Examination. A pelvic examination may detect an adnexal mass for investigation.

Ultrasound. Ultrasound is a simple tool and is usually the initial imaging examination. It helps to detect adnexal masses, although the findings are often non-specific. FT neoplasm should be considered when an unexplained solid mass is found in association with normal ovaries.

Imaging. CT or MRI can help to detect unusual tumors and to distinguish them from ovarian lesions.

Hysterosalpingography. The technique is used to confirm cases of suspected FT tumors. In such cases we frequently find a large irregular intraluminar mass.

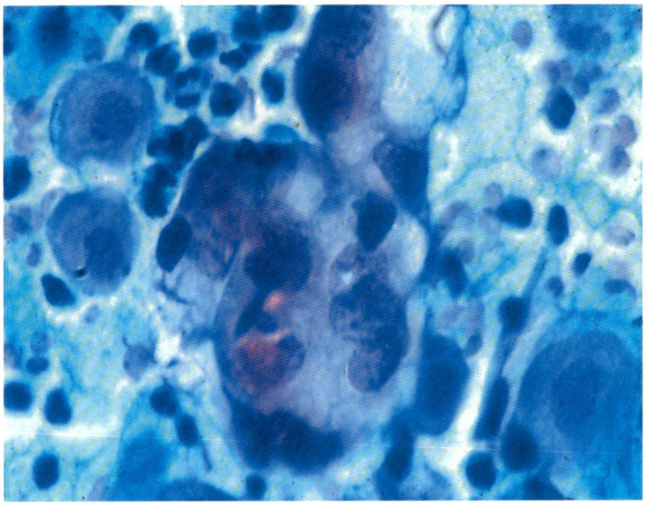

Fig. 10.4. Vaginal smear showing signs of extra-uterine adenocarcinoma. A primary tubal adenocarcinoma was subsequently found.

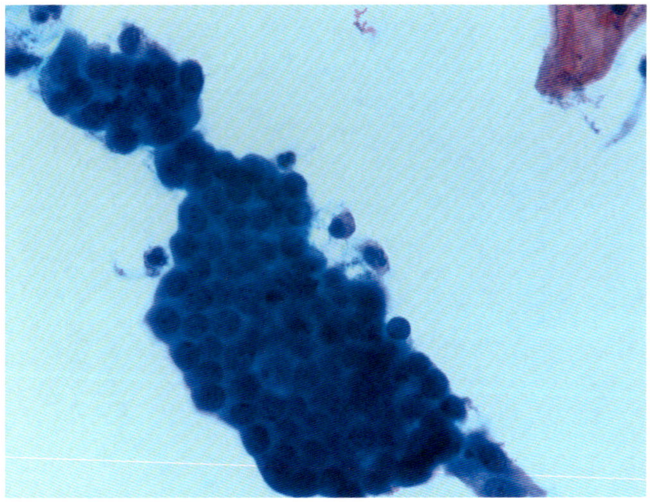

Fig. 10.5. Cytology of a prolapsed fallopian tube.

CA 125. A blood test of CA 125 is a non-specific test that tends to give elevated results in patients with FTC. It is very useful in the follow-up of tubal neoplasm, especially if there is a suspicion of recurrent carcinoma.

10.4.1. Cytology

Cervico-Vaginal Smear. This is a controversial subject. Most authors consider it an insensitive method for screening patients, although some have published good results. Takashina et al. [20] found a positive cervicovaginal smear in 37.9% of the 61 cases of primary tubal cancer with a preoperative cytologic examination.

In a few cases FTC has been diagnosed as an incidental finding of abnormal glandular cells in routine cervical smears. The possibility of FTC should be considered if cervical or endometrial cytology shows atypical glandular cells, but an endometrial or cervical primary cancer cannot be identified. Adnexal malignancy (ovary, FT) is responsible for up to 10% of cases of glandular malignant cells found in cervicovaginal or endometrial cytology. Psammoma bodies are found in some cases of well-differentiated serous carcinoma and are helpful if they are in relation with glandular malignant cells. When atypical glandular cells are found in a routine smear, further diagnostic procedures should include a repeat smear, colposcopy and hysteroscopy with endometrial biopsy. If cervical and endometrial studies are negative, ultrasound, laparoscopy and even a laparotomy should be considered. We reported a primary papillary tubal adenocarcinoma in a post-menopausal patient with sporadic vaginal bleeding (fig. 10.4) [10]. A vaginal smear showed signs of extra-uterine adenocarcinoma whereas dilatation and curettage produced insufficient material.

Vaginal cytology is useful in the follow up of patients diagnosed with tubal malignancy [11].

Endometrial Aspiration. It may be possible to collect some fluid content from the FT, despite the absence of endometrial invasion. This seems capable of giving a good diagnostic yield [11].

Ascitic Fluid and Peritoneal Washing. These are only occasionally helpful in the diagnosis. The utility of peritoneal washing cytology in the identification of occult malignancy has been documented [14].

10.4.2. Cytological Features

- Clear background. Paucity of cellular material.
- Cells. Smears usually show glandular cells, single or in papillary clusters. If the cytology suggests adenocarcinoma but the morphology is unusual for an endocervical or endometrial adenocarcinoma, an extrauterine tumor should be considered or a post-hysterectomy adenocarcinoma [21].
- FTC should be suspected when malignant cells are found in patients with unremarkable pelvic examination, negative endometrial curettage, and negative ultrasound and hysteroscopy examination [9].

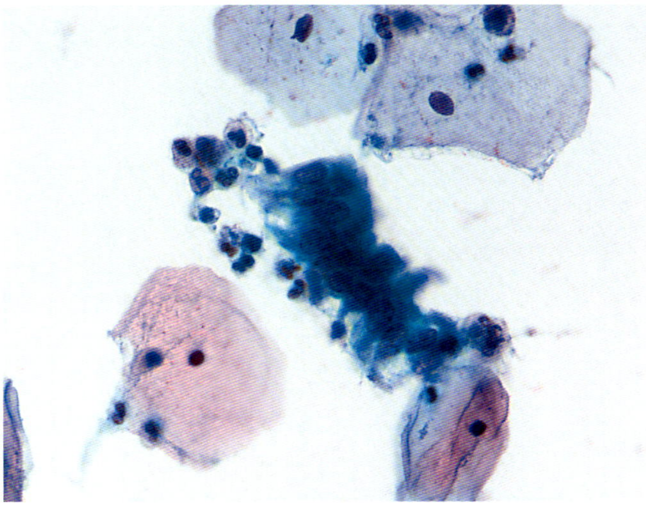

Fig. 10.6. Cytology of a prolapsed fallopian tube. Cilia are easily seen and give an important clue to the diagnosis.

10.5. Differential Diagnosis

From the point of view of the cytological differential diagnosis, it is important to distinguish between FTC from other adenocarcinomas of genital (ovary -ipsilateral ovary by direct invasion or contralateral ovary via peritoneal spread-, uterus) or extragenital sites (gastrointestinal tract), and with benign lesions such as the prolapse of the FT.

Prolapse of the FT. This is a rare benign process that can occur after hysterectomy with preservation of the FT. Clinically, it presents with vaginal bleeding and increased secretion. The vaginal smear shows glandular columnar cells with micro-nucleoli and cilia and an inflammatory background (fig. 10.5, 10.6). The histological findings are of granulation tissue with tubal epithelium, which could show some cellular atypia that has to be differentiated from vaginal metastasis of FTC, and from primary vaginal adenocarcinoma [18].

References

1 Alvarado-Cabrero I, Cheung A, Caduff R: Tumors of the fallopian tube: epithelial tumors; in Fattaneh A, Tavassoli FA, Devilee P (eds): Tumors of the breast and female genital tract. Lyon, IARC Press, 2003, pp 206–211.

2 Alvarado-Cabrero I, Young RH, Vamvakas EC, Scully RE: Carcinoma of the Fallopian Tube: a clinicopathological study of 105 cases with observations on staging and prognostic factors. Gynecol Oncol 1999;72:367–379.

3 Bibbo M, Wilbur DC: Comprehensive Cytopathology, ed 3. Amsterdam, Elselvier, 2008.

4 Cohen CJ, Thomas GM, Hagopian GS: Neoplasms of the fallopian tube; in Bast RC Jr, Kufe DW, Pollock RE, Weichselbaum RR, Holland JF, Frei E (eds): Holland-Frei Cancer Medicine, ed 5. Philadelphia, BC Decker, 2000.

5 Culton LK, Deavers MT, Silva E, Liu J, Malpica A: Endometrioid carcinoma simultaneously involving the uterus and the fallopian tube: a clinicopathological study of 13 cases. Am J Surg Pathol 2006; 30:844–849.

6 Daya D, Young RH, Scully RE: Endometrioid carcinoma of the fallopian tube resembling an adnexal tumor of probable wolffian origin: a report of six cases. Int J Gynecol Pathol 1992;11:122–130.

7 Fukunaga M, Bisceglia M, Dimitri L: Endometrioid carcinoma of the fallopian tube resembling a female adnexal tumor of probable wolffian origin. Adv Anat Pathol 2004;11:269–272.

8 Gray W: Carcinoma of Fallopian Tube Female Genital Tract: Diagnostic Cytopathology. Amsterdam, Elsevier, 1995, pp 817–819.

9 Goswami PK, Kerr-Wilson R, Mc Carthy K: Cancer of the fallopian tube. The Obstetrician and Gynaecologist 2006;8:147–152.

10 Guerra JM, Jiménez-Ayala M, Zomeño M, Aleman J, Saiz-Pardo F: Carcinoma primitivo de trompa diagnosticado mediante citología vaginal. Acta Ginecol 1976;29:92–101.

11 Hirai Y, Chen JT, Hamada T, Fujimoto I, Yamauchi K, Hasumi K, Masubuchi K, Sakamoto A: Clinical and cytologic aspects of primary fallopian tube carcinoma: a report of ten cases. Acta Cytol 1987; 31:834–840.

12 Hu CY, Taymor ML, Hertig AJ: Primary carcinoma of the fallopian tube. Am J Obstet Gynecol 1950;59:58–67.

13 Jackson-York GL, Ramzy I: Synchronous papillary mucinous adenocarcinoma of the endocervix and fallopian tubes. Int J Gynecol Pathol 1992;11:63–67.

14 Jorns JM, Knoepp SM: Occult fallopian tube carcinoma detected in routine pelvic washing specimen submitted for staging: another justification for pelvic washing cytology. Diagn Cytopathol 2009;37: 923–929.

15 Safret A, Bösch B, Bannwart F, Rinderknecht B, Hafner HU: Carcinoma in situ of the fallopian tube presenting as a positive Pap-smear. Acta Cytol 2004;48:462–464.

16 Sedlis A: Primary carcinoma of the fallopian tube. Obstet and Gynecol Surv 1961;16:209–226.

17 Seidman JD: Mucinous lesions of the fallopian tube: a report of seven cases. Am J Surg Pathol 1994;18:1205–1212.

18 Song YS, Kang JS, Park MV: Fallopian tube prolapse misdiagnosed as vault granulation tissue: a report of three cases. Pathol Res Pract 2005;201: 819–822.

19 Steward SL, Wike JM, Foster SL, Michau F: The incidence of primary fallopian tube cancer in the United States. Gynecol Oncol 2007;107:392–397.

20 Takashina I, Ito E, Kudo R: Cytologic diagnosis of primary tubal cancer. Acta Cytol 1985;29:367–372.

21 Warshal DP, Burgetson ER, Aikins JK, Rocerelo TF: Post-histerectomy fallopian tube carcinoma presenting with a positive Papanicolaou smear. Obstet Gynecol 1999;94:834–836.

Chapter 11

Metastatic Glandular Lesions

11.1. Introduction

Metastases (MT) to the female genital tract often present diagnostic problems for both the clinician and the pathologist. With the exception of ovarian MT, secondary tumors are so uncommon that they may be overlooked or misinterpreted in the differential diagnosis of genital tract lesions.

The largest series of MT to the female genital tract was published by Mazur et al. [25]. They compiled 325 cases from over 445,000 successive patients. The ovary and vagina were the most common locations of MT from both genital and extra-genital primaries, 27% of which were a potential source of diagnostic error. The ovary was the most common location of MT with an unexpected or unusual source.

Some metastatic lesions present clinically as secondary deposits in patients with disseminated disease, but others may be mistaken for primary neoplasms. The therapeutic implications are obvious. This chapter is devoted to metastatic glandular lesions providing some guidelines to their identification.

11.2. Metastases to the Genital Tract

Almost all of the genital tract MT are epithelial tumors, either adenocarcinoma or squamous cell carcinoma. A confident diagnosis can be made by cytology in many cases, especially if immunostaining can be performed and/or if a complete clinical history is provided. Diagnostic samples can be obtained by fine-needle aspiration cytology (FNAC) of palpable nodules of vulva or vagina, and ultrasound-guided FNAC of ovarian masses. Cancer cells may find their way to the vagina through the fallopian tubes, the endometrial cavity and the endocervical canal, therefore cervicovaginal and direct endometrial smears can also contain malignant cells, providing clues to the distinction between a primary and a secondary lesion. However, a history of a treated or co-existing malignant tumor outside of the female genital tract does not rule out a second primary tumor within the genital tract. For example, the association of mammary carcinoma with synchronous or metachronous carcinoma of the uterine cervix, endometrium, and ovaries is not uncommon.

11.2.1. Metastases to the Vulva

Vulvar MT are rare but often mimic a primary tumor. They can arise either through direct extension or by hematogenous or lymphatic spread from neoplasms of the female genital tract. The origin of the tumor can be genital – endometrium (fig. 11.1) [6, 35] or ovary (fig. 11.2) [8] – or it can be extragenital – breast (fig. 11.3) [36] or kidney [20].

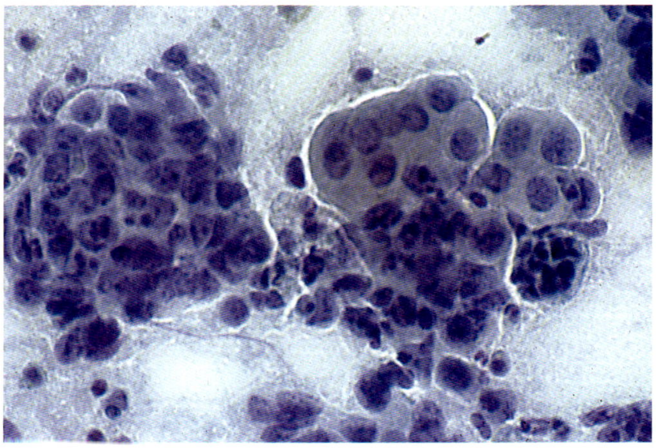

Fig. 11.1. FNA of a metastasis in vulva from an endometrial adenocarcinoma. Pap.

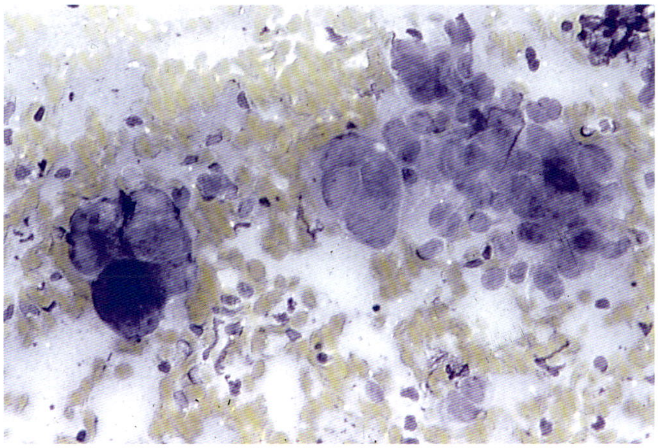

Fig. 11.2. FNA of a metastasis in vulva from an ovarian adenocarcinoma. D-Q.

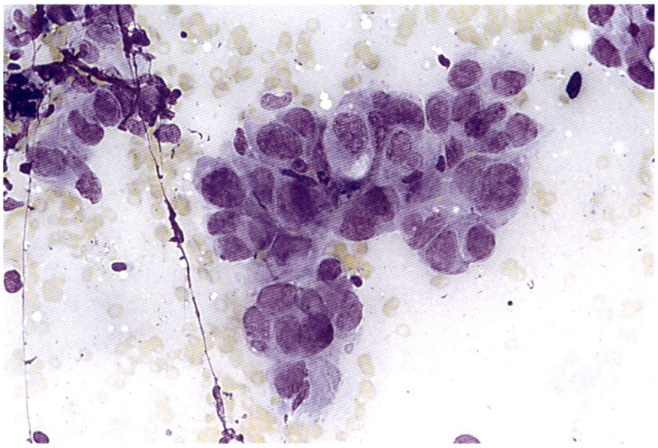

Fig. 11.3. FNA of a metastasis in vulva from a breast adenocarcinoma. D-Q.

FNAC can be very useful in the diagnosis of cutaneous or subcutaneous masses, particularly in the assessment of primary, metastatic, or recurrent malignant neoplasms. When the primary tumor is known, the MT can be rapidly and accurately diagnosed by FNAC. A combination of FNAC and immunostaining may also help define the site of an unknown primary [10, 27].

11.2.2. Metastases to the Vagina

MT to the vagina are more frequent than primary malignant tumors. The tumors may develop by direct extension, most commonly from the cervix, by vascular and lymphatic

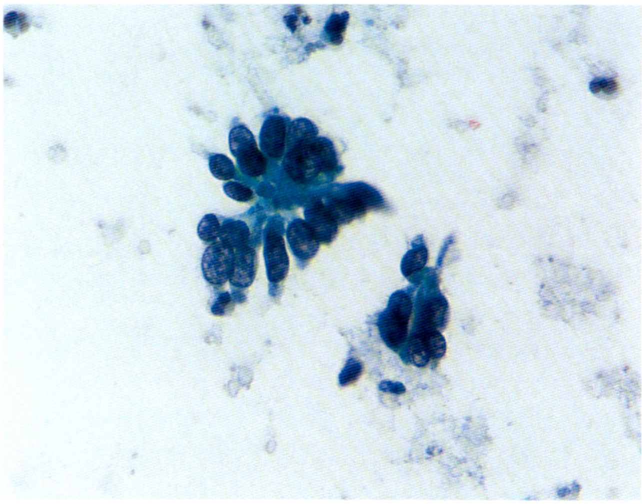

Fig. 11.4. Gland formation and a necrotic background typical from a colonic carcinoma. Pap.

permeation, or by implantation. The majority of vaginal MT from extra-genital tumors are from colorectal cancer (fig. 11.4). Direct extension from a rectal cancer to the posterior wall of the vagina is not rare, but true vaginal MT from colonic cancer is exceedingly rare. This often signals an ominous prognosis [2]. Rare primary sites such as pancreas [7] or lung [12] have been described.

Special attention has been given to vaginal clear cell adenocarcinoma (CCA) and its differential diagnosis. Primary vaginal CCA has been reported in young women who were exposed to diethylstilbestrol (DES) in the uterus. Vaginal CCA not associated with DES is very rare. More common sites of CCA in women are the ovary, endometrium, cervix, vagina and urinary tract (fig. 11.5).

Vaginal MT of renal cell carcinoma is rare, with fewer than 100 cases reported. In most cases, the vaginal lesion was detected before the diagnosis of the primary renal tumor. In practically all cases, the lesion occurs in the lower third of the vagina, most frequently on the anterior wall and toward the same side as the primary renal tumor [31]. Consequently, this tumor should be included in the differential diagnosis in all cases suspected of vaginal CCA. The diagnosis of primary clear cell carcinoma of the vagina, should be made based on a normal cytopathologic examination of the cervix, endometrium and ascites; normal appearance of the uterus, ovaries and kidneys on MRI; and absence of detectable tumor in the urinary tract [38].

Cervicovaginal cytology fails to detect most vaginal tumors. FNAC can be useful in some cases. Cytologic examination, ancillary studies, and clinical information can help

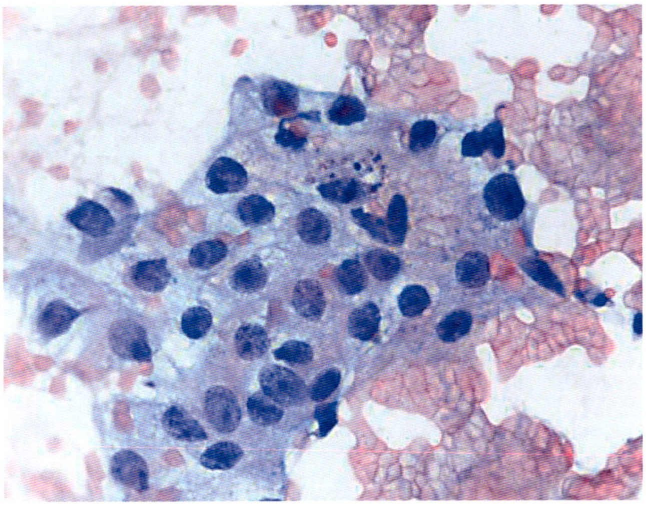

Fig. 11.5. Cytological features of clear cell carcinomas from ovary, endometrium, cervix, vagina and urinary tract are almost identical. Pap.

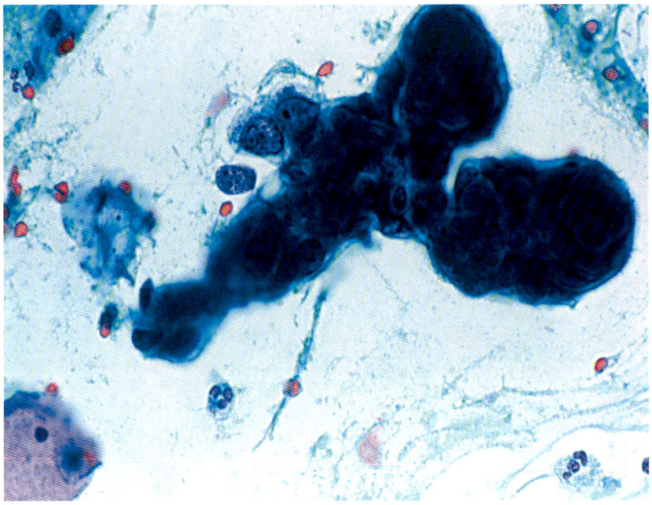

Fig. 11.7. The diagnosis of adenocarcinoma was made in a routine cervicovaginal smear, and the primitive tumor was later found in an ovary. Pap.

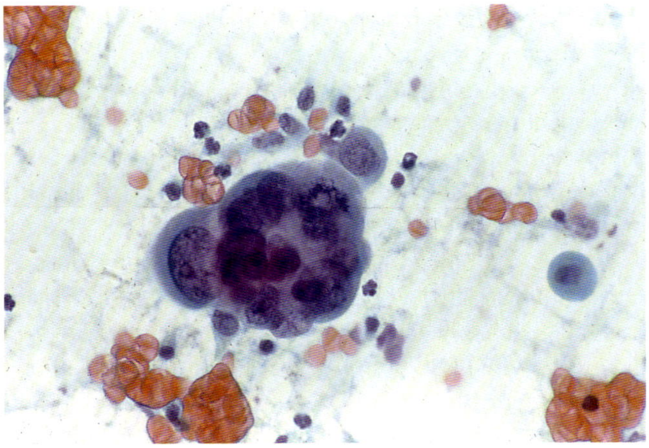

Fig. 11.6. Papilla with high-grade cells and presence of a mitosis. Follow-up showed an ovarian carcinoma metastatic to the cervix. Pap.

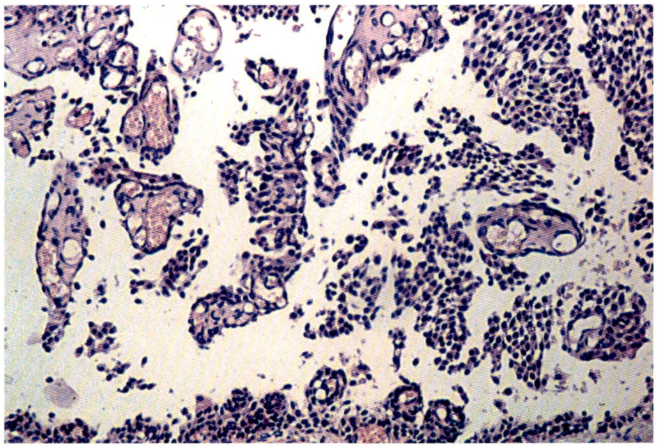

Fig. 11.8. The adenocarcinoma diagnosed in figure 11.7 was a serous surface papillary carcinoma of the ovary metastatic to a cervical polyp. Pap.

in the diagnosis and to establish the origin of the metastases [11, 27].

11.2.3. Metastases to the Cervix

Carcinoma metastatic to the cervix is very unusual. In one of the largest series published, Esposito et al. [3] reported 78 cases of extragenital carcinoma metastatic to the uterine cervix in their 1965 review of the literature. Forty-one of those carcinomas had their origin in the breast, 32 in the stomach, 4 in the lung, 2 each in the kidney, pancreas and sigmoid colon, and 1 each in the transverse colon, rectosigmoid, liver and gallbladder [3]. The ovary is the most frequent origin of intragenital MT to the cervix (fig. 11.6) [21]. MT to endocervical polyps are rare and the few cases that have been described were originated in endometrial or cervical tumors. Jiménez-Ayala described in 1996 the unique case of a serous surface papillary carcinoma (SSPC) of the ovary metastatic to a cervical polyp (fig. 11.7). The diagnosis of adenocarcinoma was made in a routine cervicovaginal smear (CVS), and the primitive tumor was later found in an ovary (fig. 11.8) [13]. SSPC is a clinicopathologic variant of ovarian carcinoma, limited to the surface or with minimal focal stromal invasion. Due to its more aggressive behavior and poorer prognosis, it should not be confused with conventional serous papillary carcinoma of the ovary.

The most frequent origin of MT to the cervix is tumors of the breast or stomach. Breast carcinoma can metastasize at any time during the long natural course of the disease, with a propensity for symptomatic MT to present many years after treatment of the primary tumor. Pambucian et al. [30] described a rare case of breast cancer initially diagnosed on a CVS. The correct interpretation of signet ring cells as metastatic, most likely from the breast or stomach, was the clue to the subsequent evaluation, and a breast biopsy finally confirmed the presence of an infiltrating lobular carcinoma [30]. Genital tract MT occur late in the evolution of breast cancer and generally are part of widely disseminated disease. Kennebeck et al. described a rare case where metastatic breast carcinoma was limited to the genital tract [18].

The incidence of gastric carcinoma in females shows a marked geographical variation and the occurrence of cervical MT has been reported mainly in oriental patients. Different cytological features have been found; the presence or absence of tumor necrosis is variable as is the size and the arrangement of the tumor cells, and the presence of nucleoli or signet-ring cells [24]. Signet-ring cells are highly suggestive of a gastric primary, but other possible sources, such as cervix, large bowel and breast, cannot be ruled out without careful consideration.

It is important to consider a metastatic tumor in the differential diagnosis of cervical adenocarcinoma in patients with an atypical presentation, and to perform a thorough work-up for metastatic disease (including immunohistochemical stains if possible) before initiating therapy. Sometimes, the primary may be found in an uncommon site such as the gallbladder [23] or the lung [16]. Sozen et al. diagnosed an adenocarcinoma in a routine CVS of a 17-year-old woman as the first finding of an asymptomatic colon cancer [33].

11.2.4. Metastases to the Endometrium

MT to the mucosal surfaces of the uterus is very uncommon, and likely to present clinically as a primary tumor. The ovary is the most frequent origin. Kumar and Schneider published 11 cases of MT to the uterus from extra-genital tumors [19]. Their experience suggests that metastatic uterine involvement must always be considered in a woman presenting with uterine bleeding and a history of previous carcinoma, in particular of breast, stomach and colon. Histologically, metastatic carcinoma of the uterus is characterized by focal involvement, lack of necrosis, and lack of accompanying premalignant changes in the endometrium, raising at least a suspicion of this entity even in the absence of a suggestive history.

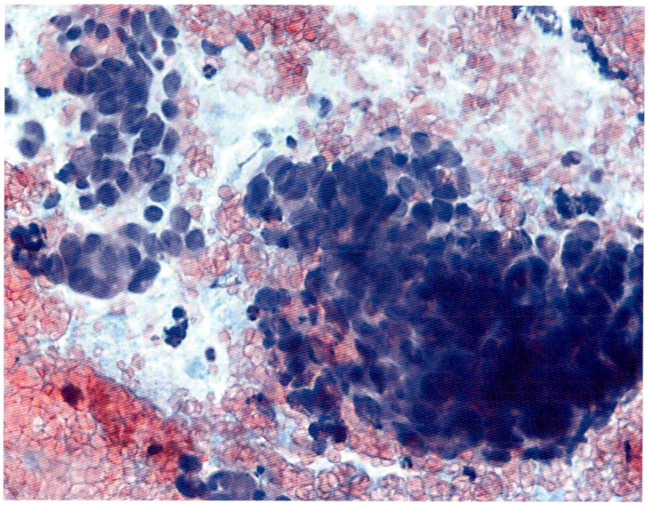

Fig. 11.9. The same extrauterine carcinoma metastatic to the endometrium as in figure 11.10 was seen in an endometrial cytology. Pap.

There are few reports on extrauterine malignancies detected by endometrial cytology (EC), and most such reports are related to ovarian cancer [34]. EC is more effective than cervical cytology for detecting cancer cells. Moreover, EC detects extragenital malignancies more often than does endometrial biopsy, because EC samples a large part of the endometrial surface (fig. 11.9, 11.10). It is therefore more likely to detect malignant cells in the uterine cavity, even if there is no endometrial invasion. Okadome et al. [29] describe 13 cases of extragenital malignant cells detected in endometrial smears performed by scraping (endocyte device). Ten of the 13 cases were diagnosed as of extrauterine origin based on the characteristic appearance of the cancer cells, the absence of cell debris associated with the poorly differentiated adenocarcinoma and, above all, the morphological difference between normal endometrial cells and cancer cells [29]. Most articles describe EC using aspiration techniques, even for preoperative diagnosis [15]

Rare cases of MT to endometrial polyps have been described [1, 17].

11.2.5. Metastases to the Ovary

The ovary is the organ where most genital MT are localized and is the most common site for unexpected MT [25].

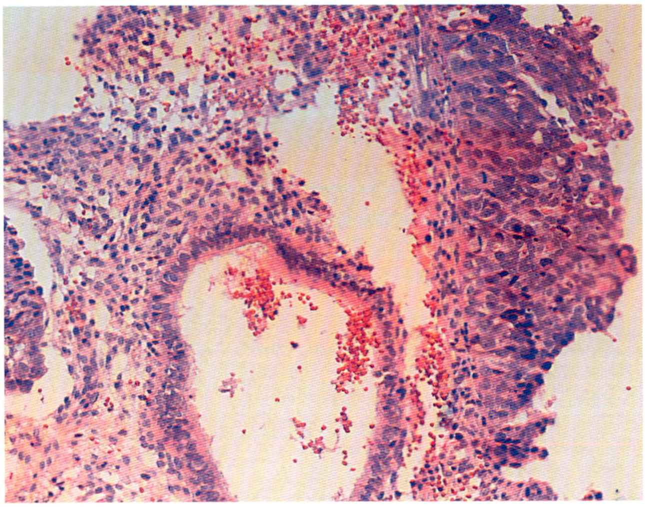

Fig. 11.10. A 70-year-old woman had a disseminated metastatic tumor of unknown origin. She died 2 months later. Endometrial biopsy. E-O.

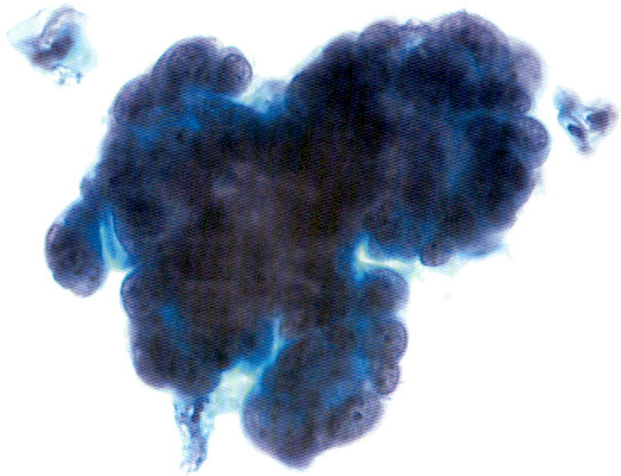

Fig. 11.11. A papillary arrangement of the malignant cells usually indicates an ovarian origin. Thin Prep. Pap.

In a large study [37], MT to the ovary accounted for 15% of all ovarian malignancies identified in a 22-year period. Among 116 patients diagnosed with MT to the ovary, the gastrointestinal tract was the most common primary site (39%), followed by breast (28%) and endometrium (20%). There were 22 MT to the ovary that mimicked a primary ovarian tumor at first clinical presentation, most of which (36%) originated from a primary tumor of the large intestine. Ovarian cysts were present in 71% of patients, and most ovaries with metastatic disease were 10 cm in diameter or less. Bilateral ovarian involvement was present in 69% of the patients, including all patients with primary tumors of the stomach.

Cytological aspects of Krukenberg tumor and other metastatic tumors to the ovary are explained in chapter 8.

11.3. Origin of Metastases

Adenocarcinoma, often poorly differentiated, is by far the most common type of metastatic malignancy, although metastatic squamous cell carcinomas, urothelial carcinomas, sarcomas, lymphomas or melanomas can also occur.

11.3.1. Intragenital Metastases

Cancers primary in one organ of the female genital tract may metastasize to another organ. For example, MT of ovarian or endometrial carcinoma to the vagina are not uncommon. The cytologic presentation is often similar to that of the primary tumor. The synchronous presentation of tumors in the endometrium and ovary needs special consideration. It is possible that 1 of the 2 neoplasms is in fact a metastasis from the other.

11.3.1.1. Metastases of Ovarian Origin

Epithelial carcinoma of the ovary accounts for approximately 75% of cases in which malignant cells that shed into the uterus, cervix or endometrium cannot be attributed to uterine cancer. A papillary arrangement of the malignant cells usually indicates an ovarian origin and is less frequently seen in endometrial, renal, urothelial, pancreatic, thyroid or mesothelial metastases (fig. 11.11). Serous papillary carcinoma of the ovary may spread from the ovary to the vagina or uterus. The cytological findings in CVS are characterized by papillary structures of malignant cells with pleomorphic macro-nucleoli, sometimes psammoma bodies (PB), and a lack of tumor diathesis.

Serous surface papillary carcinoma of the ovary (SSPC) is a distinctive clinicopathological entity within the spectrum of serous epithelial tumors, which is limited to the ovarian surface or shows minimal focal stromal invasion, and grossly unremarkable ovaries. It has a more aggressive behavior than serous papillary carcinoma (SPC) and it is more widely spread. We have published an SSPC of the ovary metastatic to a cervical polyp. To the best of our knowledge, this is the only published case of a metastasis from an ovarian tumor to a cervical polyp [13].

It seems that the identification of PB in CVS is frequently associated with malignancy of the genital tract. PB are found in less than 0.001% of consecutive screened smears, and they are associated with ovarian malignancy or ovarian borderline tumors in 22.7% of cases [4].

11.3.1.2. Metastases of Endometrial Origin

There are several types of endometrial carcinoma with different cytological features [14]. Endometrioid carcinoma is the most frequent type, but mucinous, clear cell or serous carcinomas also occur. Endometrial papillary serous carcinoma is a clinically aggressive and morphologically distinct variant of adenocarcinoma which closely resembles ovarian papillary serous carcinoma. These lesions are easily recognized by microscopic examination and typically feature a high degree of cytological anaplasia, a papillary growth pattern, and sometimes PB.

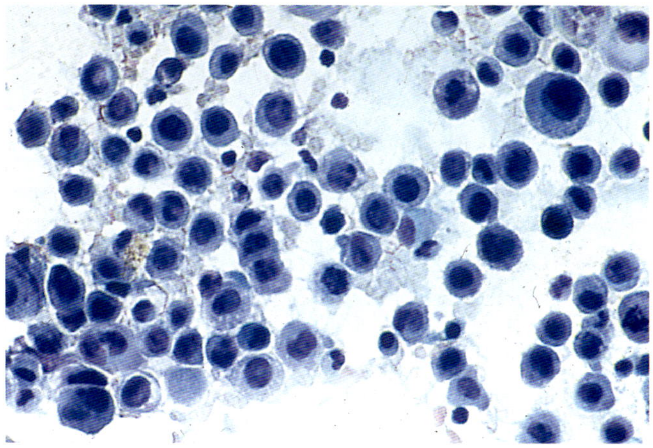

Fig. 11.12. Ascitic fluid containing malignant cells from a gastric adenocarcinoma. These cells can go through the fallopian tubes or uterus and can be seen in a cervicovaginal smear. Pap.

11.3.2. Extragenital Metastases

The female genital tract is rarely involved by metastatic disease from primary tumors of extra-genital organs. This can be a challenge for both clinicians and pathologists. There are 2 routes by which malignant cells of extragenital carcinoma can reach the cervix and appear in cytological samples. One route is direct exfoliation from the cervix, the other is the passage of ascitic fluid containing malignant cells through the fallopian tubes or uterus (fig. 11.12).

The most extensive experience to date, published by Mazur et al. [25], describes 149 cases of extra-genital MT. The primary tumor was diagnosed before or concurrently with the discovery of metastases in 80% of the cases.

11.3.2.1. Breast carcinoma

Mammary carcinoma is by far the most common source of extragenital MT to the female genital tract. Lobular carcinomas are more likely to metastasize to the genital tract than are ductal carcinomas, and are also more likely to escape clinical detection and first manifest as metastatic disease. The cytological presentation depends on the type of breast cancer, although most often, the smears contain clusters of malignant cells suggestive of adenocarcinoma without distinguishing features. Sometimes, metastatic lobular carcinoma may present with a signet-ring cell pattern or with cells in single files. The main differential diagnosis includes adenocarcinoma of endometrial, endocervical and gastrointestinal tract origin [22, 32]. On ThinPrep Pap test, the cells of lobular carcinoma show small nuclei, scant cytoplasm and more hyperchromatic nuclei than in conventional smears [7].

A few cases of metastatic breast adenocarcinoma in endometrial polyps have been published [1].

11.3.2.2. Gastrointestinal Tract

The gastrointestinal tract is one of the most important sources of ovarian MT found in surgical material [37], and can also mimic primary carcinomas of the ovary. A well-known manifestation of metastatic gastrointestinal cancer to the ovary is the Krukenberg tumor, in which signet-ring cancer cells are associated with a spindle cell reaction of the ovarian stroma. Clinical complaints related to the genital tract may be the first evidence of disease.

Carcinomas of the colon and rectum relatively frequently invade the female genital tract. In rare cases, the diagnosis of colonic cancer may be first suggested in a CVS. The cytological features of metastatic colorectal carcinoma are single cells or aggregates of columnar malignant cells with palisading or forming rosettes. The nuclei are large and the cytoplasm may be vacuolated, or less often, the cancer cells are of the signet-ring type. The differential diagnosis of colonic adenocarcinoma comprises primary adenocarcinoma of the endocervix and vaginal adenocarcinoma, the latter particularly in young women with history of maternal exposure to DES. The presence of normal endocervical cells in the smear is in favor of metastatic colonic carcinoma. Adenocarcinomas of a variety of other distant primary sites may occasionally metastasize to the female genital tract. Their exact identification is rarely possible in the absence of a clinical history. Gallbladder [17, 23], pancreas [5] and lung [12] are some of the primaries that have been reported.

11.4. Clues for the Diagnosis of Metastatic Carcinomas in Cervicovaginal Smear

A positive diagnoses of extrauterine malignancy in CVS is most likely to be made in patients who have a known, previously diagnosed primary neoplasm. The degree of tumor differentiation and the extent of tumor involvement do not appear to correlate with diagnostic yield [9]. The number of cases with malignant cells of extrauterine origin is dependent upon the frequency of CVS in the follow-up of women treated for cancer and of those suspected to have metastatic cancer. Such studies are not often done and are considered noncontributory to patient management. However, the presence of malignant cells in CVS can provide important information about the extent of the disease in these patients [28]. Esposito et al. recommended that patients with carcinoma of the breast or ovary be routinely examined for the possibility of cervical MT [3].

The main clues for the diagnosis of metastatic carcinomas (MC) in CVS are:

- MC usually exfoliate fewer abnormal cells than primary tumors. The number of abnormal cells does not correlate well with origin, histologic type, or vaginal or cervical involvement by the tumor [9].
- The importance of the presence of tumor diathesis is subject to debate. It has been stated that the CVS background in MC is often free of necrotic material and debris ('tumor diathesis'), when compared with primary carcinomas. However Gupta and Balsara [9] did not find a statistically significant association between the presence or absence of tumor diathesis in primary versus metastatic carcinoma. Inflammation, necrosis and blood may be observed in smears, particularly if MC has formed a large lesion with a necrotic surface.
- PB are a rare finding in CVS (fig. 11.13). For some authors, the presence of PB in normal CVS of asymptomatic women is an incidental finding [26] while for others, this finding should not be ignored and should generate clinical investigation to identify its source, especially in old women and/or patients with clinical symptoms such as postmenopausal bleeding [4]. In general, the most reliable predictor of malignancy for smears containing PB is the finding of cells in the CVS that by themselves are cytologically diagnostic of malignancy. PB are generally associated with papillary serous carcinomas, most frequently of ovarian origin, but sometimes of the endometrium. PB have been described in benign processes such as infections or intrauterine contraceptive devices.

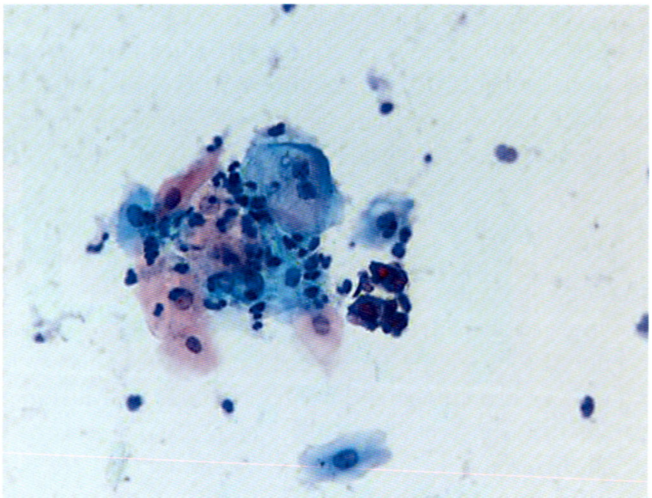

Fig. 11.13. Psammoma bodies are generally associated with papillary serous carcinoma, most frequently of ovarian origin, but they have also been described in benign processes or as an incidental finding. Pap.

- When adenocarcinoma is identified in a CVS, an extrauterine primary should be considered if tumor cells are scant and unevenly distributed in the smear. The cells have generally larger nuclei and less vacuolated cytoplasm than those of endometrial adenocarcinoma, and phagocytosis is rare. Cytological and histological endometrial specimens present benign endometrial findings [14].
- The diagnosis of MC can be suspected when the malignant cells are not consistent with any of the known patterns of cancer of the female genital tract.
- Some architectural or cytological aspects can provide clues to the possible origin of the tumor. Papillary groups suggest an ovarian origin, but endometrial, renal cell, pancreatic carcinomas or mesotheliomas cannot be excluded. Cells in single file suggest breast or gastric cancer. Intracytoplasmic lumina strongly suggest breast cancer and a signet-ring pattern suggests an origin from stomach or breast. Clear cells are highly suspicious of renal cell carcinoma and tall cells with cigar-shaped nuclei, especially if associated with necrosis and 'terminal bars' are indicative of a colorectal carcinoma (fig. 11.14).

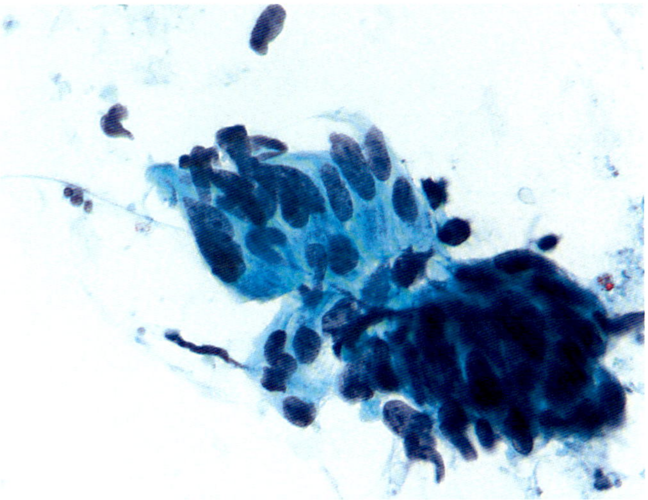

Fig. 11.14. Tall cells with cigar-shaped nuclei, especially if associated with necrosis and 'terminal bars' are indicative of a colorectal carcinoma. Pap.

As a final remark, MT to the female genital tract is rare and their clinical evolution is usually insidious. The clinical detection and diagnosis of MT often precedes the diagnosis of the primary tumor. For this reason, it is very important to consider a metastatic tumor in the differential diagnosis in patients with an atypical presentation of adenocarcinoma in order to avoid diagnostic and therapeutic errors. A thorough work-up including immunohistochemical stains if possible, should be performed. When MT appear in the female genital tract the survival rate is generally poor as it implies wide dissemination of the tumor in a short period of time [25].

References

1 Al-Brahim N, Elavathil LJ: Metastatic breast lobular carcinoma to tamoxifen-associated endometrial polyp: case report and literature review. Ann Diagn Pathol 2005;9:166–168.
2 Chagpar A, Kanthan SC: Vaginal metastasis of colon cancer. Am Surg 2001;67:171–172.
3 Esposito JM, Zarou DM, Zarou GS: Extragenital adenocarcinoma metastatic to the cervix uteri. Am J Obstet Gynecol 1965;92:792–795.
4 Fadare O, Chacho MS, Parkash V: Psammoma bodies in cervicovaginal smears: significance and practical implications for diagnostic cytopathology. Adv Anat Pathol 2004;11:250–261.
5 Fader AN, Brainard JA, Rose PG: Symptomatic vaginal bleeding in a postmenopausal woman: a case report of pancreatic adenocarcinoma metastasizing exclusively to the vagina. Am J Obstet Gynecol 2007;197:e8–e9.
6 Giordano G, Gnetti L, Melpignano M: Endometrial carcinoma metastatic to the vulva: a case report and review of the literature. Pathol Res Pract 2005; 201:751–756.
7 Green KM, Turyan HV, Jones JB, Hoda RS: Metastatic lobular carcinoma in a ThinPrep Pap test: cytomorphology and differential diagnosis. Diagn Cytopathol 2005;33:58–59.
8 Guidozzi F, Sonnendecker EW, Wright C: Ovarian cancer with metastatic deposits in the cervix, vagina, or vulva preceding primary cytoreductive surgery. Gynecol Oncol 1993;49:225–228.
9 Gupta D, Balsara G: Extrauterine malignancies: role of Pap smears in diagnosis and management. Acta Cytol 1999;43:806–813.
10 Gupta RK, Naran S: Fine needle aspiration cytology of cutaneous and subcutaneous metastatic deposits from epithelial malignancies: an analysis of 146 cases. Acta Cytol 1999;43:126–130.
11 Hughes JH, Jensen CS, Donnelly AD, Cohen MB, Silverman JF, Geisinger KR, Raab SS: The role of fine-needle aspiration cytology in the evaluation of metastatic clear cell tumors. Cancer 1999;87: 380–389.
12 Jahnke A, Domke R, Makovitzky J, Nizze H, Briese V: Vaginal metastasis of lung cancer: a case report. Anticancer Res 2005;25:1645–1648.
13 Jiménez-Ayala M, Martínez Cabruja R, Esteban ML, Chinchilla C: Serous surface papillary carcinoma of the ovary metastatic to a cervical polyp: a case report. Acta Cytol 1996;40:765–769.
14 Jiménez-Ayala M, Jiménez-Ayala Portillo B: Endometrial Adenocarcinoma: Prevention and Early Diagnosis. Monogr Clin Cytol. Karger, Basel, 2008, vol 17.
15 Jobo T, Arai M, Iwaya H, Kato Y, Ohno E, Kuramoto H: Usefulness of endometrial aspiration cytology for the preoperative diagnosis of ovarian carcinoma. Acta Cytol 1999;43:104–109.
16 Kai K, Takai N, Nasu K, Kira N, Ishii T, Kashima K, Narahara H: Metastatic uterine cervical cancer originating in the lung: a case report. Gynecol Obstet Invest 2009;68:269–271.
17 Kefeli M, Gonullu G, Can B, Malatyalioglu E, Kandemir B: Metastasis of adenocarcinoma of the gall bladder to an endometrial polyp detected by endometrial curettage: case report and review of the literature. Int J Gynecol Pathol 2009;28:343–346.
18 Kennebeck CH, Alagoz T: Signet ring breast carcinoma metastases limited to the endometrium and cervix. Gynecol Oncol 1998;71:461–464.
19 Kumar A, Schneider V: Metastases to the uterus from extrapelvic primary tumors. Int J Gynecol Pathol 1983;2:134–140.
20 Leiman G, Markowitz S, Veiga-Ferreira MM, Margolius KA: Renal adenocarcinoma presenting with bilateral metastases to Bartholin's glands: primary diagnosis by aspiration cytology. Diagn Cytopathol 1986;2:252–255.
21 Lemoine NR, Hall PA: Epithelial tumors metastatic to the uterine cervix: a study of 33 cases and review of the literature. Cancer 1986;57:2002–2005.
22 Mallow DW, Humphrey PA, Soper JT, Johnston WW: Metastatic lobular carcinoma of the breast diagnosed in cervicovaginal samples: a case report. Acta Cytol 1997;41:549–555.
23 Martínez-Román S, Frumovitz M, Deavers MT, Ramirez PT: Metastatic carcinoma of the gallbladder mimicking an advanced cervical carcinoma. Gynecol Oncol 2005;97:942–945.
24 Matsuura Y, Saito R, Kawagoe T, Toki N, Sugihara K, Kashimura M: Cytologic analysis of primary stomach adenocarcinoma metastatic to the uterine cervix. Acta Cytol 1997;41:291–294.
25 Mazur MT, Hsueh S, Gersell DJ: Metastases to the female genital tract: analysis of 325 cases. Cancer 1984;53:1978–1984.
26 Muntz HG, Goff BA, McGonigle K, Isacson C: The significance of psammoma bodies in screening cervical cytologic smears. Am J Obstet Gynecol 2003;188:1609–1612; discussion 1612–1614.

27 Nadji M, Defortuna S, Sevin BU, Ganjei P: Fine-needle aspiration cytology of palpable lesions of the lower female genital tract. Int J Gynecol Pathol 1994;13:54–61.

28 Ng ABP, Teeple D, Linder EA, Reagan JW: The cellular manifestations of extrauterine cancer. Acta Cytol 1974;18:108–117.

29 Okadome M, Saito T, Tsukamoto N, Nishi K, Nishiyama N, Nagata E: Endometrial scraping cytology in women with extragenital malignancies. Acta Cytol 2006;50:158–163.

30 Pambuccian SE, Bachowski GJ, Twiggs LB: Signet ring cell lobular carcinoma of the breast presenting in a cervicovaginal smear: a case report. Acta Cytol 2000;44:824–830.

31 Queiroz C, Bacchi CE, Oliveira C, Carvalho M, Rabelo Santos D: Cytologic diagnosis of vaginal metastasis from renal cell carcinoma: a case report. Acta Cytol 1999;43:1098–1100.

32 Rau AR, Saldanha P, Raghuveer CV: Metastatic lobular mammary carcinoma diagnosed in cervicovaginal smears: a case report. Diagn Cytopathol 2003;29:300–302.

33 Sozen I, Small L, Kowalski M, Mayo SW, Hurwitz CA: Adenocarcinoma of the cervix metastatic from a colon primary and diagnosed from a routine pap smear in a 17-year-old woman: a case report. J Reprod Med 2005;50:793–795.

34 Takashina T, Ono M, Kanda Y, Sagae S, Hayakawa O, Ito E: Cervicovaginal and endometrial cytology in ovarian cancer. Acta Cytol 1988;32:159–162.

35 Temkin SM, Hellman M, Lee YC, Abulafia O: Surgical resection of vulvar metastases of endometrial cancer: a presentation of two cases. J Low Genit Tract Dis 2007;11:118–121.

36 Valenzano Menada M, Papadia A, Lorenzi P, Fulcheri E, Ragni N: Breast cancer metastatic to the vulva after local recurrence occurring on a rectus abdominis myocutaneous flap: a case report and review of the literature. Eur J Gynaecol Oncol 2003;24:577–579.

37 de Waal YR, Thomas CM, Oei AL, Sweep FC, Massuger LF: Secondary ovarian malignancies: frequency, origin, and characteristics. Int J Gynecol Cancer 2009;19:1160–1165.

38 Watanabe Y, Ueda H, Nozaki K, Kyoda A, Nakajima H, Hoshiai H, Noda K: Advanced primary clear cell carcinoma of the vagina not associated with diethylstilbestrol. Acta Cytol 2002;46:577–581.

Chapter 12

Ancillary Techniques for the Diagnosis of Glandular Lesions of the Female Genital Tract

12.1. Introduction

The ancillary techniques applied on cytology of female genital tract glandular lesions have been developed almost exclusively in those of the endocervix and for differential diagnoses between the endocervix and endometrium. Consequently we focus here on endocervical lesions.

Endocervical glandular lesions are rare, benign cases, which are much more frequent than malignant ones. Benign lesions may be classified into several groups: (1) metaplasia, including tubal, endometrial or tubulo-endometrial cases; (2) hyperplasia, such as 'tunnel clusters'; (3) endocervical lobular hyperplasia, diffuse or microglandular; (4) decidual change, such as the Arias Stella Reaction; (5) endometriosis, and (6) embryological remnants, such as mesonephric remnants, including hyperplastic and neoplastic changes, as well as prostatic remnants.

The most important lesions are obviously those which are neoplastic and preneoplastic. From the histological point of view, they may be classified as adenocarcinoma in situ (AIS) or endocervical adenocarcinoma, with all the histological variants. Both lesion types – in situ and infiltrating – have their corresponding cytological pictures. However, so-called 'precursor' lesions, such as atypical glandular cells (fig. 12.1; glandular endocervical dysplasia, which has been classified by some authors into low- or high-grade cervical glandular intraepithelial neoplasia, including in situ adenocarcinomas), may correspond to neoplastic or reactive histological lesions.

On the other hand, the relationship between human papilomavirus (HPV) infection and neoplastic endocervical lesions is well known. In around half of the reported glandular neoplastic cases, HPV infection and its relationship to glandular and squamous lesions explain the coexistence of both lesions in the same patient.

There is little experience with or consensus on the utilization of complementary cytological techniques with respect to the glandular lesions. This could be due to the fact that they are not as frequent as squamous lesions and also because they are more heterogeneous.

In the cervicovaginal smears of uterine glandular lesions, 2 problems are usually encountered. First, we need to decide if the observed atypia is the result of an existing HPV infection and, therefore, an indication of the risk of a preneoplastic or neoplastic cervical lesion. Second, the origins of atypical cells are not always obvious, since in a cervicovaginal smear we may encounter endocervical, endometrial, ovarian, tubal or metastatic cells. It is helpful to apply the morphological criteria recommended by the Bethesda System, but for the clinician, as well as the pathologist, there always exists some level of uncertainty when dealing with the diagnosis of glandular atypia.

The atypia of endocervical cells is frequently associated with the squamous lesions caused by HPV, both low and high grade, and on fewer occasions glandular atypia is the only lesion present in the cytology. In these cases, it is helpful to attempt to discover the origin of the glandular cells. When dealing with endocervical cells, the decision of whether the atypia is responsive to reactive phenomena or is truly a preneoplastic lesion is very important. Cytological diagnosis has been substantially refined in the last decade and pathologists can now better recognize the cytological representation of AIS. However, as always in morphology, there exists a gray zone in which complementary techniques can be of great value, such as may be observed in the case of squamous lesions (atypical squamous cells of undetermined significance).

The detection of preneoplastic or neoplastic lesions in the biopsy following a cytological diagnosis of atypical glandular cells is sufficiently frequent that most clinical guides recommend performing a colposcopy and biopsy after such a cytological diagnosis. Approximately 30% of these patients have disease, most of them high- and low-grade squamous lesions with a low percentage (3%) presenting with AIS and approximately 5% with adenocarcinomas, most of which are of endometrial origin. It is clear that when dealing with this situation, cytopathologists should reserve this diagnosis for when they truly believe that a fundamental risk of these types of lesions exists.

The establishment of a score for evaluating glandular endocervical lesions has been attempted, which would result in an increase in the interobserver reproducibility for non-invasive glandular endocervical lesions in histological samples, including stratification, atypia, mitosis and apoptosis. Criteria are given scores between 0 and 3 (counting upwards). When comparing the scores 6–9 against the rest, the coincidence is 95%. This score does not have an application in cytology.

The ancillary techniques that can help us to identify malignant endocervical lesions in cytological samples are similar to those used for squamous lesions: the HPV probe, immunohistochemical procedures for p16 and others.

12.2. HPV Probe

HPV determination may be performed using hybrid capture or PCR methods.

12.2.1. Hybrid Capture II

Second-generation hybrid capture (HC2) is a standardized and robust, FDA-approved method with high sensitivity for endocervical adenocarcinoma, similar to the probe for high-grade squamous cervical lesions.

The HC2 HPV DNA test is a nucleic acid hybridization assay with signal amplification using microplate chemiluminescence for the quantitative detection of 18 low- and high-risk types of HPV in cervical specimens. These specimens contain target DNA hybrids, which are revealed using a specific HPV RNA probe. The resultant RNA DNA hybrids are captured onto the surface of a microplate, which is well-coated with antibodies specific to those RNA DNA hybrids. The immobilized hybrids are then reacted with alkaline phosphatase-conjugated antibodies specific to the RNA-DNA hybrid and detected using a chemiluminescent substrate. A substance signal permits semi-quantitative measurement. This method provides information on the viral DNA in the specimens and also a on the viral load (fig. 12.1).

This method uses 2 classes of probes that identify low- and high-risk HPV DNA. The high-risk types detected are 16, 18, 31, 33, 35, 39, 45, 51, 56, 58, 59 and 68; and the low-risk types are 6, 11, 42 and 43. However, in practice many laboratories use only the high-risk types.

A large number of clinical studies have proved the sensitivity, specificity and reproducibility of this technique as a primary screening method for the general population. Its use is common in many countries. It has shown the HC2 test is more effective than conventional Pap smears in the primary screening of patients with adenosquamous carcinoma of the cervix (ASC), due to its greater sensitivity and identical specificity. In the follow-up of patients after excisional treatment, this test offers high sensitivity for lesion reappearance offering, along with the Pap smear, the best specificity available.

However, this method does not allow us to distinguish between the different viral types or between multiple infections. When cells of the atypical glandular type are detected in cytology, a positive result for HPV using the HC2 technique is of great value for reaffirming the risk of glandular or squamous histological lesions. The positive predictive value is similar to that of squamous lesions, and the sensitivity for the detection of endocervical adenocarcinoma is high. However, if the atypical cells have their origin in endometrial or ovarian lesions, the usefulness of the HPV test is clearly nullified. For this reason, as in cases of ASC, a negative HPV test has a great negative predictive value for lesions. For glandular atypia, however, this predictive value is not enough. For this and other reasons, some authors believe that when faced with a glandular lesion with a negative HPV result, it is advisable to repeat the test [1–12].

12.2.2. PCR

PCR methods may also be used. Ideally, a specialized laboratory with specialized technicians is needed, in order to test the various specimens using different consensus primers, in order to be sure of their positivity and/or negativity. However, this technique is not currently accepted by the FDA. PCR allows the typification of the virus and multiple infections (fig. 12.2). Recently, a series of standards have been developed to validate diverse techniques for HPV detection, as compared to Hybrid Capture techniques.

	1	2	3	4	5	6	7	8	9	10	11	12
A ID RLU Ratio Result	Outlier NC 102	10V335 36 0.10 --	10V343 32 0.09 --	10V351 54978 167.61 Low Risk	10V359 29 0.08 --	10V367 38 0.11 --	NC 70	10V335 1013862 3417.47 High Risk	10V343 1470 4.95 High Risk	10V351 224 0.75 --	10V359 46 0.15 --	10V367 116 0.39 --
B ID RLU Ratio Result	NC 64	10V336 42 0.12 --	10V344 64 0.19 --	10V352 17162 52.32 Low Risk	10V360 68 0.20 --	10V368 48 0.14 --	NC 58	10V336 10158 34.24 High Risk	10V344 58 0.19 --	10V352 858021 2892.17 High Risk	10V360 514689 1734.88 High Risk	10V368 68 0.22 --
C ID RLU Ratio Result	NC 56	10V337 48 0.14 --	10V345 34 0.10 --	10V353 3504 10.68 Low Risk	10V361 60 0.18 --	10V369 174 0.53 --	NC 82	10V337 1724 5.81 High Risk	10V345 42 0.14 --	10V353 66 0.22 --	10V361 18966 63.92 High Risk	10V369 90442 304.85 High Risk
D ID RLU Ratio Result	LRC 324	10V338 72 0.21 --	10V346 32 0.09 --	10V354 29 0.08 --	10V362 36 0.10 --	10V370 44 0.13 --	HRC 306	10V338 50 0.16 --	10V346 98 0.33 --	10V354 72 0.24 --	10V362 84 0.28 --	10V370 195696 659.64 High Risk
E ID RLU Ratio Result	LRC 344	10V339 34 0.10 --	10V347 36 0.10 --	10V355 3812 11.62 Low Risk	10V363 68 0.20 --	10V371 34 0.10 --	HRC 298	10V339 46 0.15 --	10V347 5068 17.08 High Risk	10V355 243967 822.35 High Risk	10V363 50 0.16 --	10V371 46 0.15 --
F ID RLU Ratio Result	LRC 316	10V340 34 0.10 --	10V348 25 0.07 --	10V356 54 0.16 --	10V364 32 0.09 --	10V372 40 0.12 --	HRC 286	10V340 440 1.48 High Risk	10V348 34 0.11 --	10V356 44 0.14 --	10V364 242 0.81 --	10V372 720 2.42 High Risk
G ID RLU Ratio Result	QC1-LR - V 1222 3.72 Valid	10V341 33 0.10 --	10V349 66 0.20 --	10V357 31 0.09 --	10V365 52 0.15 --	10V373 34 0.10 --	QC1-LR - V 68 0.22 Valid	10V341 38 0.12 --	10V349 80124 270.07 High Risk	10V357 42 0.14 --	10V365 164 0.55 --	10V373 852 2.87 High Risk
H ID RLU Ratio Result	QC2-HR - V 154 0.46 Valid	10V342 34 0.10 --	10V350 32 0.09 --	10V358 34 0.10 --	10V366 72 0.21 --	10V374 32 0.09 --	QC2-HR - V 1252 4.22 Valid	10V342 1616 5.44 High Risk	10V350 42 0.14 --	10V358 48652 163.99 High Risk	10V366 84594 285.14 High Risk	10V374 40 0.13 --

DIGENE

Hybrid Capture® II Software v.2.0
Instrument Serial #: 2432

Supervisor: ______________________ Date: ______________

Fig. 12.1. Hybrid Capture II. Results: number of specimens and viral load.

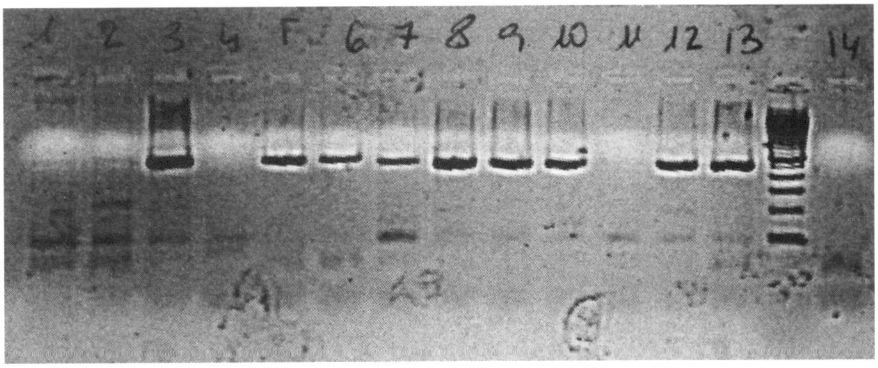

Fig. 12.2. HPV PCR, using MYO primers. Bands 1–12: Problem cases. Band 14: Positive and negative controls.

12.3. Immunohistochemical Techniques for p16 [13, 14]

When faced with a cytological lesion classified as having atypia of the glandular cells, immunoreactivity for p16 (fig. 12.3) can slant the diagnosis towards a lesion suspected of malignancy. Endocervical adenocarcinomas are very frequently immunoreactive for p16 (fig. 12.4). However, endometrial adenocarcinoma can also be immunoreactive for

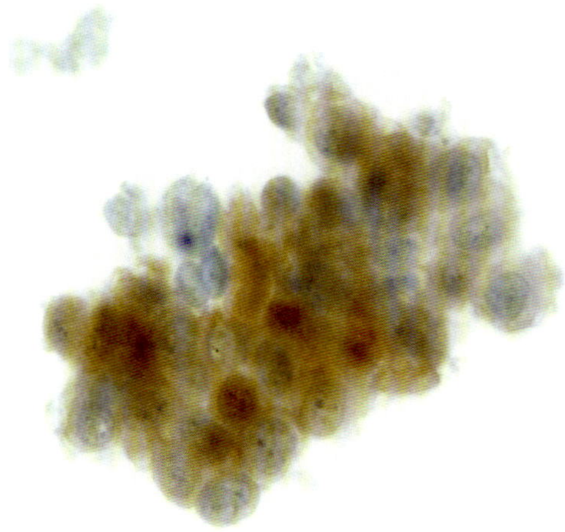

Fig. 12.3. Atypical glandular cells. Cytology. Cells p16+ and p16–.

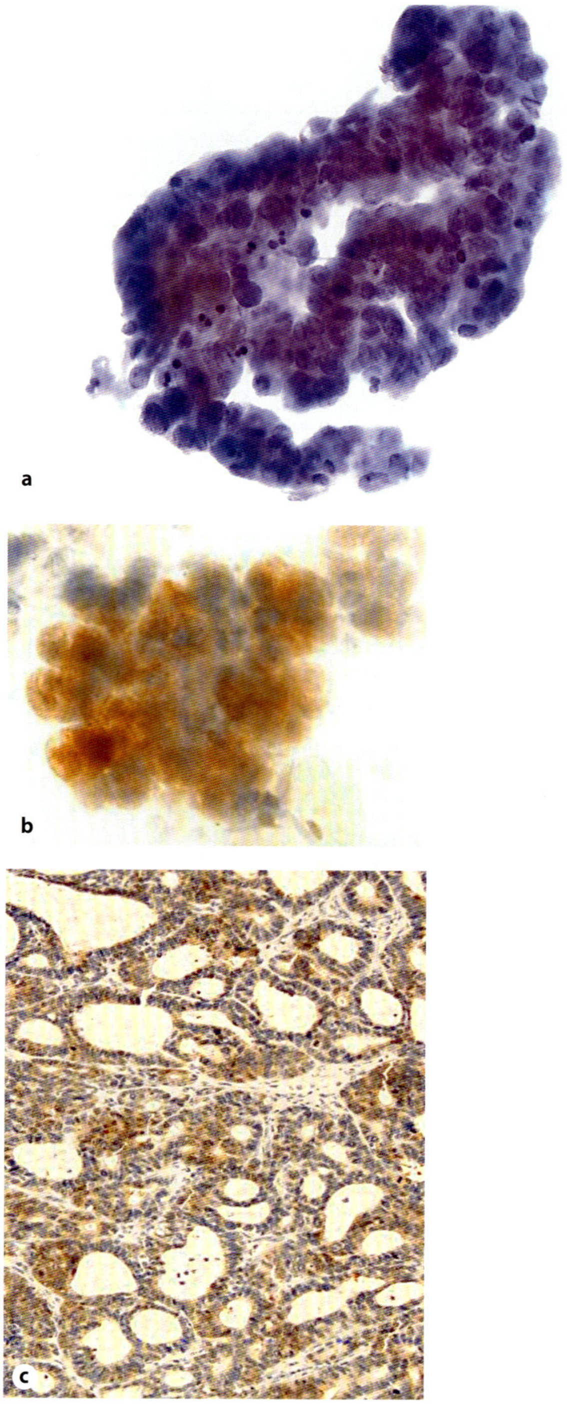

Fig. 12.4. Endocervical adenocarcinoma. **a** Cytology. **b** Cytology. Cells p16+. **c** Histology. p16+.

p16 (fig. 12.5), as with squamous cell carcinoma and malignant mixed Müllerian tumors (fig.12.6). For this reason, the immunoreactivity for p16 in a glandular lesion suspected of malignancy can lean towards the diagnosis of a malignant lesion. However, histogenetic typification cannot be based solely on immunoreactivity for p16, since some authors have shown that in histological samples the extension of the reaction has clarified the localization of the same (nuclear or nuclear and cytoplasmic versus cytoplasmic). This can be utilized as an orienting fact with regards to the endocervical or endometrial origins of a lesion.

Immunocytochemical detection of the over-expression of protein p16 (MTM Laboratories), which is characteristic of high-risk HPV infections that have already provoked a dysfunction in the regulation of the cellular cycle by the action of the oncogenic proteins E6 and E7, is not easy in cytological cases of glandular atypia, due to the non-specific staining observed in normal and metaplastic glandular cells. A typical example is that of tubal metaplasia. It must be remembered that this entity provides a differential diagnosis of glandular atypia, which is also frequently positive for p16. Though the histological pattern in the staining of a bona fide glandular atypia is relatively simple to discern, in cytology it is not so clear. In order to consider a dysplastic glandular lesion suspicious, it is not only important to appraise the positivity of the p16 staining in the glandular cells, but the nuclear and/or architectural atypia should also be observed.

Recently, a commercial kit for cervicovaginal samples has been developed that joins p16 and ki67 immunoreactivity in the same cell (p16 = brown; ki67 = red), allowing both

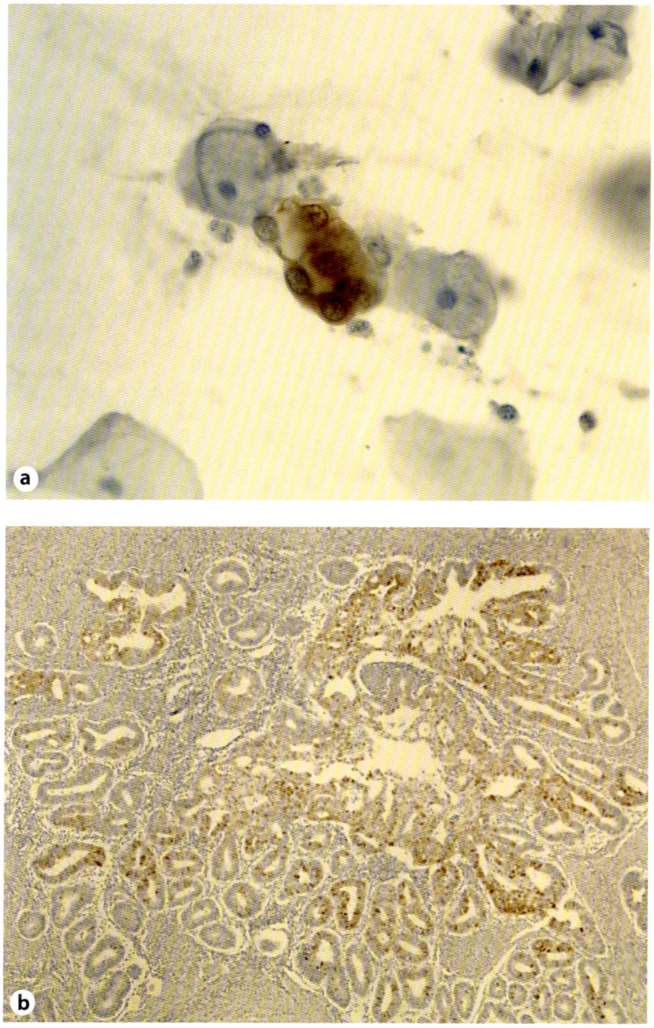

Fig. 12.5. Endometrial adenocarcinoma. **a** Cytology. Cells p16+. **b** Histology. p16+.

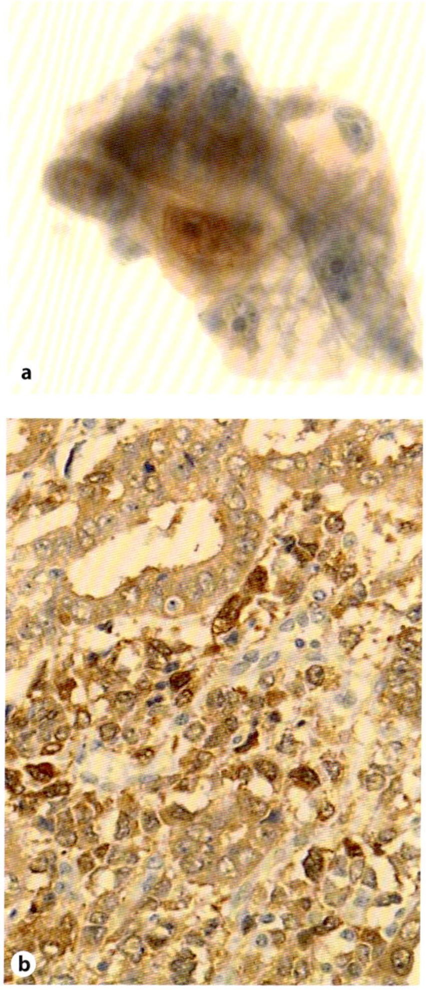

Fig. 12.6. Malignant mixed Müllerian tumor. **a** Cytology. Cells p16 + and p16–. **b** Histology. p16 + in both epithelial and mesenchymal components.

to be evaluated in a single double-stained cell (fig. 12.7). Under these conditions, the test shows high sensitivity (similar to HC2 test), and high specificity (greater than HC2) for CIN2+. This kit can be used in both conventional and liquid-based cytology.

12.4. Other Techniques

There is another immunocytochemical stain for detecting the simultaneous over-expression of topoisomerase II alpha (TOP2A) and the MCM2 protein (ProExC). Though in the literature there are scant data, it seems that its usefulness in cases of ASC is similar to that of p16, in that it detects the cells exhibiting errors in the control of cellular proliferation. It is possible that the staining described in normal endocervical cells also makes interpretation difficult in the diagnosis of glandular atypia [15, 16].

Immunohistochemical techniques for BCL2 and Ki67 can be useful in distinguishing between benign and malignant lesions, and immunohistochemical techniques for estrogen receptors, progesterone receptors, Vimentin, and carcinoembrionic antigen can help to distinguish between endocervical and endometrial lesions, though they are not usually applied in cytology.

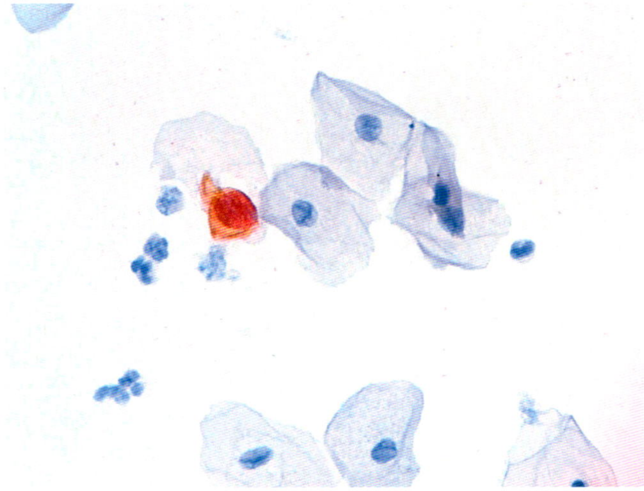

Fig. 12.7. CINtec Plus+. p16 stains the cytoplasm in brown and ki67 stains the nucleus in red.

12.5. Conclusion

In summary, when faced with the discovery of glandular atypia along with suspicion of endocervical lesions, we can make an extrapolation of the data obtained using the existing techniques for squamous lesions of the cervix (HPV, p16) knowing that, in this case, the sensitivity is good. However, we should keep in mind that endometrial lesions, frequently associated with this diagnosis, will not benefit from the techniques commented on above. In addition, it is possible for errors to be made in immunocytochemical interpretation. Given the high incidence of serious lesions (30%) associated with a diagnosis of glandular atypia, most authors recommend that a colposcopy, hysterectomy and/or endocervical curettage be carried out immediately.

References

1 Arbyn M, Buntix F, Van Ranst M, Paraskevaidis E, Martin-Hirsch P, Dillner J: Virology versus cytology triage of women with equivocal pap smears: a meta-analysis of the accuracy to detect high grade intraepithelial neoplasia. J Natl Cancer Inst 2004;96:280–293.

2 Barreth D, Faught W, Schepausky A, Johnson G: The relationship between atypical glandular cells of undetermined significance on Pap smear and a clinically significant histologic diagnosis. J Obstet Gynaecol Can 2004;26:867–870.

3 Chen L, Yang B: Assessment of reflex HPV DNA testing in patients with atypical endocervical cells on cervical cytology. Cancer 2008;114:236–241.

4 Han CP, Kok LF, Wang PH, Wu TS, Tyan YS, Cheng YW, Lee MY, Yang SF: Scoring p16INK4 immunohistochemistry based an independent nuclear staining alone can sufficiently distinguish between endocervical and endometrial adenocarcinomas in a tissue microarray study. Modern Pathol 2009; 22:797–806.

5 Ioffe OB, Sagae S, Moritani S. Dahmoush L, Chen TT, Silverberg SG: Proposal of a new scoting scheme for the diagnosis of noninvasive endocervical glandular lesions. Am J Surg Pathol 2003;27: 452–460.

6 Ioffe OB, Sagae S, Moritani S. Dahmoush L, Chen TT, Silverberg SG: Symposium part 3: should pathologists diagnose endocervical preneoplastic lesions 'less than' adenocarcinoma in situ? Int J Gynecol Pathol 2003;22:18–21.

7 Levine L , Lucci JA 3rd, Dinh TV: Atypical glandular cells: new Bethesda terminology and management guidelines. Obstet Gynecol Surv 2003;58: 399–406.

8 McCluggage WG: Endocervical glandular lesions: controversial aspects and ancillary techniques. J Clin Pathol 2003;56:164–173.

9 Mejier, C JLM, Berkhof J, Castle PE, Hesselink AT, Franco EL, Ronco G, Arbyn M, Bosch FX, Cuzik J, Dillner J, Heideman DAM, Snijders PJF: Guidelines for human papillomavirus DNA requirements for primary cervical cancer screening in women 30 years and older. Int J Cancer 2009; 124:516–520.

10 Mulvany NJ, Allen DG, Wilson SM: Diagnostic utility of p16INK4a: a reappraisal of its use in cervical biopsies. Pathology 2008;40:335–344.

11 Negri G, Rigo B, Vittadelo F, Mian C, Egarter-Vil E: Abnormal cervico-vaginal cytology with negative human papillomavirus testing. Cancer (Cancer Cytopathol) 2007;111:280–284.

12 Ronnett BM, Manos MM, Ransley JE, Fetterman BJ, Kinney WK, Hurley LB, Ngai JS, Kurman RJ, Sherman ME: Atypical glandular cells of undetermined significance (AGUS): cytopathologic features, histopathologic results, and human papillomavirus DNA detection. Hum Pathol 1999;30: 816–825.

13 Schnatz PF, Guile M, O'Sullivan DM, Sorosky JL: Clinical significance of atypical glandular cells on cervical cytology. Obstet Gynecol 2006;107: 701–708.

14 Shroyer KR, Homer P, Heinz D, Singh M: Validation of a novel immunocytochemical assay for topoisomerase ii-a and minichromosome maintenance protein 2 expression in cervical cytology. Cancer Cytopathol 2006;108:324–330.

15 Tambouret RH. Misdraji J, Wilbur DC: Longitudinal clinical evaluation of a novel antibody cocktail for detection of high-grade squamous intraepithelial lesions on cervical cytology specimens. Arch Pathol Lab Med 2008;132: 918–925.

16 Yemelyanova A, Vang R, Seidman JD, Gravitt PE, Ronnet BM: Endocervical adenocarcinomas with prominent endometrial or endomyometrial involvement simulating primary endometrial carcinomas: utility of HPV DNA detection and immunohistochemical expression of p16 and hormone receptors to confirm the cervical origin of the tumors. Am J Surg Pathol 2009;33:914–924.

Index